Crucible is published quarterly by Hymns Ancient & Modern Ltd.
Registered Charity No. 270060

This publication is in collaboration with the Church of England's
Division of Mission and Public Affairs; the William Temple Foundation.

Editorial board
Stephen Platten, Edward Cardale, Kate Pearson, Elaine Graham,
Malcolm Brown, Chris Swift, Carol Wardman,
Matt Bullimore, James Woodward, Peter Scott, Andrew Hayes
(Reviews Editor) and Anna Lawrence (Managing Editor).

Correspondence and articles
Correspondence and articles for submission should be sent to
Anna Lawrence at Hymns Ancient and Modern, anna@hymnsam.co.uk.
Articles should be of about 3,000 words.
Books for review to should be sent to Dr Andrew Hayes,
The Queen's Foundation, Somerset Road, Birmingham, B15 2QH.

Subscriptions
(for four copies): individual rate £22; institutions £30;
international (includes airmail) £40. Single copies cost £7.
All prices included postage and packing. Cheques should
be made payable to Crucible, and sent to: Crucible subscriptions,
Subscription Manager, 13a Hellesdon Park Road, Norwich NR6 5DR.

Tel: 01603 785 910   Fax: 01603 624483.
crucible@hymnsam.co.uk

Direct Debit forms available from the same address

ISSN 0011-2100
ISBN 978-0-334-05964-6

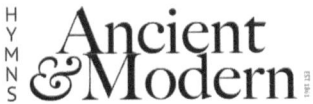

Editorial

Neil Messer   03

Articles

Ritual Impurity and Disease: 07
Reflections on Biblical 'Analogies' in the COVID Era
Justin Harrison Duff

Resilience in a Time of COVID-19 – Three Biblical Models: 16
Plague, Uncleanness and Indigestion
Megan Warner

Paschal Simultaneity in Time of Pandemic: 24
A Liturgical Theological Response to COVID-19.
Ann Swailes

A Theological Engagement with T. S. Eliot's *The Waste Land*   32
in the Context of COVID-19
Andrew Picard and Jaimee van Gemerden

Virtual Communion, COVID-19, and the Nature of   40
the Body of Christ
Hannah Bowman and Neil Dhingra

Pre-Pandemic Ethics: 49
Triage and Discrimination
Margaret B. Adam and David L. Clough

Book Reviews   57

*Beth Dodd, Martin Kettle, Jonathan Dean, Cathy Ross,
Christopher Swift*

Editorial

Pandemic Theology: Christian Theology in the Midst of COVID-19

NEIL MESSER

This issue of *Crucible* presents six articles arising from one of the earliest theological responses in the UK to the COVID-19 pandemic. In mid-March 2020, as the UK went into lockdown in response to the pandemic, I wondered aloud on Facebook what the calling of theologians was at such a time. My question provoked a livelier response than anything else I have posted on social media, and from this emerged the online conference *Christian Theology in the Midst of COVID-19*. The conference took place in June 2020, with 20 paper presentations and around 120 participants from diverse church and academic contexts around the world.

The focus was deliberately on 'first thoughts' from the midst of the pandemic. Theologians are not always known for rapid responses, but there were good reasons for beginning the work of theological reflection on the pandemic quickly, while the crisis was still unfolding. Christians and churches had to make immediate responses in their pastoral care, their worship, and their ethical and social engagement, and it was important for such responses to be theologically resourced. Ill-judged and potentially harmful religious comment on the pandemic was not slow to emerge from various quarters, and so there was a need for more considered and critical theological perspectives. But over and above these considerations, it seemed (and still seems) worth capturing some first theological thoughts from the midst of the crisis. While some questions may be better considered from a safe distance, others will come into sharper focus in the midst of things, and it is important to put on record the insights gained in this way.

A selection of six of the conference papers, revised in the light of the conference discussion, are presented in the present issue. (Earlier

Editorial

versions of most of the conference papers are available at www.winchester.ac.uk/pandemictheology.) Together they represent a cross-section of the topics addressed at the conference and the theological reflections that have emerged thus far – all of which have a bearing in various ways on Christian practices of worship, pastoral care and ethical, social and political engagement.

For those seeking scriptural perspectives on COVID-19, biblical images of plague and contagion have an obvious attraction, but some of these connections are – to say the least – questionable. Our collection begins with two papers offering critical perspectives on such uses of biblical texts. Justin Duff interrogates the superficially attractive connection between biblical texts about 'leprosy' and the modern experience of infectious disease. He argues that this connection is misleading, because these texts do not refer to what we know as leprosy (Hansen's disease), or indeed any infectious disease. They are concerned with ritual impurity, not infection in the modern sense, and we run various risks by connecting the two over-hastily – not least, stigmatizing the hundreds of thousands of people around the world who live with Hansen's disease.

Next, Megan Warner draws on her own and others' research on the Bible and trauma to seek biblical themes and models that might promote resilience in the face of COVID-19. She rejects biblical accounts of divinely-ordained plagues and of 'leprosy' as models of the pandemic. Instead she argues that an understanding of the earth itself as an agent with its own God-given vocation can be a fruitful source of narratives to help reframe our experiences of the pandemic and foster resilience in the face of trauma.

COVID-19 has raised familiar questions about how to make theological sense of suffering, and the next two papers address these questions in different ways. In dialogue with the late mediaeval authors Julian of Norwich and William Langland, Ann Swailes offers an approach based on the traditional Christian understanding that by baptism we are incorporated into Christ. Because of this, our sufferings can become a participation in Christ's suffering and saving work. This perspective has its dangers, as Swailes acknowledges, but she argues that by seeing the suffering of the cross in the light of the resurrection and vice versa, we can achieve a balanced theological perspective on suffering, avoiding both an unhealthy fascination with it and the temptation to deny or dismiss it.

Andrew Picard and Jaimee van Gemerden take up the discussion of suffering and hope in dialogue with a very different literary text: T. S. Eliot's poem *The Waste Land*. Reading Eliot's poem alongside the work of theologians Donald MacKinnon and Karen Kilby, the authors explore themes including tragedy, meaninglessness and the limits of theological talk of hope. They caution against speaking too glibly of Christ's victory or too knowingly about future hope, concluding: 'We cannot offer robust assertions of meaning regarding suffering in COVID-19, but we are invited to see that Christian hope is found in Christ's presence in and through suffering, and not aside from it.'

The final two papers more directly address questions of Christian practice in worship, ethics and politics. Hannah Bowman and Neil Dhingra take up a question that preoccupied many churches as countries around the world went into lockdown and places of worship were closed: is a virtual Eucharist possible? In this paper they continue what began as an online dialogue between them. They continue to disagree about the possibility of virtual Eucharist, but agree that this is a theological, not merely a technical, question. Drawing on Jürgen Moltmann's account of the forsakenness of Jesus on the cross, they reflect on the experience of 'absence' in a virtual Eucharist. They also observe that this absence draws attention to the absence of those excluded from public worship in 'normal' times.

Margaret Adam and David Clough begin with a question of medical ethics that preoccupied many people early in the pandemic: how should life-saving health care resources be allocated when there are insufficient for all the patients who need them? In an earlier essay Adam and Clough addressed this question and argued for an approach, in emergency situations only, aimed at saving the most lives. In the present article, however, they shift the focus away from such 'pandemic ethics' to what they call 'pre-pandemic ethics'. They describe the pandemic as an 'apocalypse': it uncovers the pre-existing systemic injustices that have made BAME people, people with disabilities and older people in care homes (for example) more vulnerable to COVID-19. Christians, they argue, should be working now to dismantle these injustices before the next pandemic.

Taken together, these six essays represent a rich vein of initial reflection on COVID-19, in which the study of biblical texts and core themes of Christian theology both inform and are informed by Christian practices of worship, pastoral care and social and political engagement. These 'first thoughts' are offered as starting points for the further reflection and action that must begin now and continue in

Editorial

the months and years ahead.

I end with a few words of thanks. When I began planning the conference, I invited Rachel Muers, Peter Scott and Chris Southgate to form a programme committee. In the midst of busy lives made busier by the pandemic, all three were kind enough to say yes, and have been extraordinarily generous with their time and expertise in reviewing paper proposals, planning and running the conference and acting as a peer-review college for this journal issue. Neither the conference nor the journal issue would have been possible without their help. Thank you to Edward Cardale, Editor of *Crucible*, for responding so enthusiastically to the idea of this theme issue and for his support and guidance as we have put it together. My thanks also to the presenters and participants who helped make the conference a fascinating and productive event, and especially to the authors of the papers in this issue, for working within tight editorial timescales to produce such rich and varied resources for thought and action.

Neil Messer is Professor of Theology at the University of Winchester.

Ritual Impurity and Disease

Reflections on Biblical 'Analogies' in the COVID Era

Justin Harrison Duff

Introduction

In the midst of global disaster, Jewish and Christian communities often turn to the pages of the Hebrew Bible for reflection, inspiration, humour, and instruction. In the COVID era, the biblical themes of social distancing, quarantine, and ritual impurity have become recurrent sources for further recollection and reading. It has become especially common to summon the biblical laws addressing 'disease' and 'quarantine' and 'isolation' in recent months. Biblical instructions concerning the quarantine and isolation of 'leprosy' (hereafter *'lepra'* when speaking of the biblical condition)[1] has become a particularly pronounced theme in a number of recent news articles, essays, and posts covering the COVID crisis.

For instance, the Wikipedia entry on 'Social Distancing'—which has been updated with a lengthy discussion of COVID-19—opens with a citation of Leviticus 13.46, the isolation instructions pertaining to persons afflicted with *lepra*. As awareness of the coronavirus grew in late January, Eleanor Klibanoff (2020) wrote an NPR article on the history of quarantine and similarly cited Leviticus 13.54 as an example of an ancient text requiring the quarantine of a 'possibly sick person.' Stephen Moss's subsequent Guardian article in late February (Moss, 2020) also cited the Levitical laws, describing ancient 'leprosy' as a 'disease' that was isolated and traced by Israel's priests. The emerging commentary on COVID-19 suggests that Levitical purity texts, like recent government instructions, were oriented around the confinement and control of persons afflicted with a contagious disease in order to stem the spread of infection.

This interpretation is also reflected amongst recent articles and essays written by religious scholars and specialists of biblical and rabbinic literature. Rabbi Dr. Jay Michaelson, for instance, addressed the COVID crisis and its intersection with humanity's 'biblical' and 'primal' terrors of disease and contagion in mid-March (Michaelson, 2020). His article in the *Daily Beast* opened with a citation of Leviticus 13.46 and indicated that persons diagnosed with *lepra* and irregular sexual discharges, persons he describes as 'sick and infirm' and 'diseased,' were isolated from the 'healthy' in the ancient world. He concludes by comparing the strict legislation surrounding biblical 'impurity' with modern fears of 'plague.' Similarly, Oxford mathematician and Christian apologist John C. Lennox, in his recently published book on God and the coronavirus (Lennox, 2020, p. 50), appeals to the Levitical laws while discussing 'The Difference God Makes' and 'Heeding Advice.' Lennox promotes 'quarantine' for contemporary persons with 'underlying medical conditions' with reference to the quarantine laws of Leviticus, which, in his view, are concerned with the 'spread of infectious illnesses.'

Yitzhaq Feder, a specialist in ancient Near Eastern purity laws, also summoned the background of Levitical impurity and *lepra* in his late-March academic essay addressing the novel coronavirus (Feder, 2020). Feder's past research (e.g. Feder, 2016; Feder, 2019) suggests that fear of contagious disease may form much of the historical background for the Levitical purity taboos and *lepra* in particular. As with COVID-19, he detects a signal of humanity's longstanding avoidance of persons who are perceived as transmitting disease, or persons 'infected' or 'afflicted' with *lepra*.

What to make of this range of supposed biblical parallels? As a biblical scholar who specializes in the reception of Levitical purity and sacrifice laws in Second Temple Jewish texts and the New Testament, the recurrent biblical 'analogies' between *lepra* and the modern-day coronavirus prompt no shortage of interest, curiosity, and critical reflection. The methods of reading the biblical texts outlined above could largely be classified as incidents of 'extratextuality' that are 'experimentally-oriented' (Alkier, 2009, pp. 9–10). Ancient texts are read in the context of contemporary extratextual signs in order to draw out effects of meaning produced by the juxtaposition. Since these reading events circulate around significant questions regarding disease and divine law, the relationship between ritual impurity and medical disease, and *lepra* and COVID-19, they warrant further reflection and investigation with an eye towards a critical theological analysis of the Mosaic laws.

Leprosy and COVID-19

There are several issues that immediately arise when comparing biblical *lepra* to COVID-19. First, comparisons of this sort are likely fueled by certain linguistic 'leprosy' metaphors that abound in the Western cultural imagination (Edmon, 2006, pp. 110–42; Sontag, 1989). Indeed, the sociological and metaphoric use of the term 'leper' with reference to persons who have tested positive for COVID-19— or are imagined to be potent vectors for the disease—has become commonplace in recent months. For instance, as recently as late May, Italian foreign minister Luigi Di Maio told the world not to treat Italy 'like a leper colony' while considering summer destinations.

The persistent use of this metaphor, however, is profoundly problematic. Leprosy proper (i.e. Hansen's disease) remains a highly stigmatized medical illness that continues to affect hundreds of thousands of persons worldwide, especially in India. Indeed, Leprosy Mission International (2020) has recently covered the significant challenges posed by the novel coronavirus to communities of persons suffering from Hansen's disease in locked-down India. As Siân Arulanantham, head of Programmes Coordination at the England and Wales branch of The Leprosy Mission, has reiterated (Mudge, 2020):

> Whenever there is a new outbreak of a disease, like the Coronavirus, I always fear the entirely inaccurate comparison with leprosy. My heart did sink when I read the inevitable headline that the 'Coronavirus is the new leprosy'. It just re-emphasises the unnecessary fear and stigma surrounding leprosy…It is only fear, ignorance and a lack of access to healthcare that sees the world's oldest disease remain a 21st Century disease.

Thus, at a minimum, one must be extremely cautious of the profound sociological impact of drawing on a biblical condition like *lepra* to explain or elucidate contemporary illnesses. Zachary Gussow (1989) has warned that uncritical comparisons of this sort were precisely the sort of moves that 'retainted' leprosy in the late nineteenth century.

Similarly, in a recent essay, Rod Edmon (2020) has highlighted the racist and panic-based parallel between Donald Trump's descriptions of the worldwide contagion as 'the Chinese virus' and descriptions of Hansen's disease on the island of Molokai in the late nineteenth-century, where the disease became racially inscribed as 'the Chinese evil.' Imperial powers have long exoticized and stigmatized contagious diseases by associating them with foreigners perceived as threats to an errant yet carefully maintained sense of national identity.

On the other hand, the recurrent historical confinement of persons who suffered from various diseases of the skin in the ancient and modern world activates certain striking parallels with the contemporary situation. Pam Fessler, for instance, has drawn some of these parallels in a recent NPR article (Fessler, 2020). But what is the *Levitical* quarantine and isolation of persons diagnosed with *'lepra'* all about? What are the purity laws communicating through their various quarantines and 'contact tracings'? To address these questions, I first discuss what biblical *lepra* is and is not, and then clarify the primary concern of the *lepra* legislation.

Lepra and biblical texts

In Leviticus and Numbers, *lepra* describes a visible condition of human skin, fabrics, and walls. *Lepra* is diagnosed by curious 'marks' of a specific colour and depth. For a 'mark' (e.g. swelling, spot, scab, boil, or burn) to be classified as *'lepra'* of the skin, it must be 'deeper' than the skin and change the colour of the hair on the surface of the skin (if there is any hair to change). Similarly, for a 'mark' to be classified as the *'lepra'* of a house, it must appear 'deeper than the walls' and be reddish or greenish in colour. For a 'mark' to be classified as *'lepra'* on a garment, it must affect the front and back of the garment and similarly present as reddish or greenish. In short, the mark must appear to be seriously decomposing a body or surface, even if it is not.

A possible case of *lepra* requires 7–14 days quarantine of the person, garment, or house. The quarantine period is required to see if the marks worsen into 'scaly marks' (*lepra*/ṣāraʿat means 'scaly' or 'dusty' or 'sandy'). These marks are not disgusting or, as Jacob Milgrom notes, 'repulsive', but instead denote 'neutral' skin conditions that are absent 'aesthetic' commentary (Milgrom, 1991, p. 775). If scales appear, the person is isolated outside the camp until the scales dissipate and the body begins to heal (Lev 13.45–46; Num 12; 2 Kgs 7).

As a result, ancient *lepra* and modern-day leprosy are dramatically different. To put it bluntly, the biblical phenomenon is not modern-day Hansen's disease (Milgrom, 1991, p. 816; Douglas, 1999, pp. 182–83; Edmon, 2006, pp. 5–6). Hansen's disease is closer to the ancient disorder termed *elephantiasis* (*graeca*) and was probably not introduced into the Middle East until the Hellenistic Period (Milgrom, 1991, pp. 816–17). As Milgrom discusses, the closest parallels to *lepra* in the modern world are probably psoriasis and vitiligo (1991, pp. 816–17). Not even these diseases, however, comprehensively account for the details of the texts at hand.

Strikingly, much like psoriasis and vitiligo, biblical *lepra* is not contagious. The *ritual impurity* generated by *lepra* is contagious, but the underlying disease is not. And this contagious impurity, as Jonathan Klawans notes, is impermanent and removed through routine ritual procedures like water ablutions (Klawans, 2000, pp. 22–26). The cause of Hansen's disease, long thought to be hereditary, was proven to be a very mildly contagious bacteria (*Mycobacterium leprae*) in the mid-nineteenth century. Conversely, *lepra* is not treated as contagious by the priestly texts, Second Temple texts, or Jesus of Nazareth (Mark 1.40–44, Matt 8.1–3, Luke 5.12–14). Priests are required to inspect and diagnose the affliction without any sort of physical shielding or protection. Likewise, the extensive purification instructions that appear in Leviticus 14 are required for a body already healed of *lepra* (cf. further Luke 17.11–14).

Other biblical texts also suggest that *lepra* is noncontagious (e.g. Lev 14.36, 2 Kgs 5; cf. Milgrom, 1991, p. 817). A striking indicator also appears in Lev 13.12–13, which addresses *lepra* that covers the entire human body:

> If, however, the *lepra* breaks out on the skin so that the *lepra* covers all the skin of the person with the mark from his head to his feet, as far as the priest can see, the priest must then examine it, and if the *lepra* covers his whole body, he is to pronounce the person with the infection pure. It has turned all white, so he is pure.[2]

Contra modern expectations, a person covered head-to-toe with *lepra* is considered 'clean' or 'pure' in the biblical legislation. The person is free to live in their personal home, walk around communal space, congregate with family and friends, and approach the sanctuary. Thus, the biblical texts are not obsessed with the transmission of the affliction through human contact. *Lepra* is a visible condition that finds parallels across skin, fabric, and plaster. What, then, is the primary concern of the purity laws?

As with impurity in other systems, the driving concerns are not medical. Mary Douglas has argued at length that 'medical materialism' is a 'prosaic' approach to these and other ancient purity laws (Douglas, 1966, pp. 36–44, esp. p. 36). She stresses the importance of thinking back to a time before germ theory and modern society's close link between dirt and pathogen (1966, p. 44). Douglas notes that ancient dirt or impurity is better classified as 'matter out of place' (1966, pp. 44–50). Thus: 'Where there is dirt there is system' (1966, p. 44). Douglas's symbolic approach to the purity laws has become widely adopted in biblical scholarship, and often yields readings that are more profitable than those focused on 'medical' rationales.

The purity laws appear to be united by the following: *the address of conditions that symbolize the human body's subjection to the cycle of birth and death* (Milgrom, 1991, pp. 732–33, 819–20, 1002–3; Harrington, 2004, pp. 92–93; for the cycle of birth cf. Maccoby, 1999, pp. 49–50). Along with the quarantine or isolation of persons diagnosed with *lepra*, decaying garments and houses, new mothers, persons who touch a corpse, and men and women with irregular sexual discharges are confined to different degrees (Num 5.2–3, Lev 12). The connection between birth/death and parturient women and corpses is clear, and *lepra* is often likened to physical death across biblical and Second Temple texts (e.g. Num 12.12, Job 18.13–23, 4QDa). As Milgrom notes, the laws therefore communicate that God's holiness 'represents the forces of life' (1991, p. 1003), and it demands life from those who approach the sanctuary.

The Mosaic purity laws therefore appear to remind the reader that Israel's God is a God of bewildering life and evaluates the human condition from a higher gradation of staggering holiness in the local sanctuary. A close theological reading of the purity laws further reveals profound indications of God's preference for life over death. Israel's God is a thrice holy God of life who resides among chosen persons amidst their fraught, mortal existence. Thus, the purity laws are not obsessed with the containment and treatment of medical disease. Instead, their concern with contagious impurity — not contagious diseases like COVID-19 — signals the divine concern with life and highlights the astonishing, life-giving quality of God's inexorable holiness.

> *Justin Harrison Duff is a Postdoctoral Research Fellow in the Logos Institute of Analytic and Exegetical Theology at St Mary's College, University of St Andrews.*

Questions for Discussion

1. How does a disease like COVID-19 differ from biblical *lepra*?

2. What appears to be the unitive symbolic logic of the biblical purity laws?

References

Alkier, S. (2009). 'Intertextuality and the Semiotics of Biblical Texts,' in Hays, RB., Alkier, S., and Huizenga, LA., (eds.) *Reading the Bible Intertextually*. Waco, TX: Baylor University Press, pp. 3–21.

Douglas, M. (1966, repr. 2002). *Purity and Danger: An Analysis of the Concepts of Pollution and Taboo*, London: Routledge and Kegan Paul, repr., London: Routledge Classics.

Douglas, M. (1999). *Leviticus as Literature*, Oxford: Oxford University Press.

Edmon, R. 2006, *Leprosy and Empire: A Medical and Cultural History*, Cambridge Social and Cultural Histories, Cambridge: Cambridge University Press.

Edmon, R. (2020). 'Leprosy Demonstrates How Fears of Disease Spread—and then Live Forever,' March 19 [online]. Available at: httpsa//www.zocalopublicsquare.org/2020/03/19/fear-of-disease-leprosy-coronavirus/ideas/essay (Accessed: 14 August 2020).

Feder, Y. (2016). 'Defilement, Disgust, and Disease: The Experiential Basis of Hittite and Akkadian Terms for Purity,' *Journal of the American Oriental Society*, 136, pp. 99–116.

Feder, Y. (2019). April, 'Tum'ah: Ritual Impurity or Fear of Contagious Disease?', April [online]. Available at: https://www.thetorah.

com/article/tumah-ritual-impurity-or-fear-of-contagious-disease (Accessed: 14 August 2020).

Feder, Y. (2020). 'Coronavirus: What We Can Learn from the Bible and the ANE,' March 18 [online]. Available at: https://www.thetorah.com/blogs/coronavirus-what-we-can-learn-from-the-bible-and-the-ane (Accessed: 14 August 2020).

Fessler, P. (2020). February 7, 'Lessons from Leprosy For Coronavirus: Quarantine and Isolation Can Backfire,' 7 February [online]. Available at: https://www.npr.org/sections/health shots/2020/02/07/803533167/lessons-from-leprosy-for-coronavirus-quarantine-and-isolation-can-backfire (Accessed: 14 August 2020).

Gussow, Z. (1989). *Leprosy, Racism, and Public Health: Social Policy in Chronic Disease Control*. New York: Avalon Publishing.

Harrington, H. K. (2004). *The Purity Texts, Companion to the Qumran Scrolls 5*. London: T&T Clark.

Klawans, J. (2000). *Impurity and Sin in Ancient Judaism*, Oxford: Oxford University Press.

Klibanoff, E., (2020). 'A History of Quarantines, From Bubonic Plague to Typhoid Mary, January 26 [online]. Available at: https://www.npr.org/sections/goatsandsoda/2020/01/26/799324436/a-history-of-quarantines-from-bubonic-plague-to-typhoid-mary (Accessed: 14 August 2020).

Lennox, J. C. (2020). *Where is God in a Coronavirus World?* Epsom: The Good Book Company.

Leprosy Mission International (2020). 'How are People Affected by Leprosy Coping with the Biggest Lockdown in the World?', 1 May [online]. Available at: https://www.leprosymission.org/our-story/blog/detail/our-blog/2020/05/01/how-are-people-affected-by-leprosy-coping-with-the-biggest-lockdown-in-the-world (Accessed: 14 August 2020).

Maccoby, H. (1999). *Ritual and Morality: The Ritual Purity System and its Place in Judaism*. Cambridge: Cambridge University Press.

Michaelson, J. (2020). 'The Biblical, Primal Terror of the Coronavirus,' 10 March [online]. Available at: https://www.thedailybeast.com/the-dangerous-primal-terror-of-the-coronavirus (Accessed: 14 August 2020).

Milgrom, J. (1991). *Leviticus 1–16: A New Translation with Introduction and Commentary, Anchor Bible 3*. New York: Doubleday.

Moss, S. (2020)., 'From the Black Death to Coronavirus: a Brief History of Quarantines,' February 26 [online]. Available at: https://www.

theguardian.com/world/shortcuts/2020/feb/26/coronavirus-quarantines-brief-history-contain-epidemics (Accessed: 14 August 2020).

Mudge, H. (2020). 'Stigmatised Travelers Exposed to the Coronavirus Quarantined at Former Leprosy Asylum that Remains Home to Those Bearing the Scars of the Ancient Disease,' 6 March [online]. Available at: https://www.leprosymission.org.uk/latest-news/stigmatised-travellers-exposed-coronavirus-quarantined-former-leprosy-asylum-remains-home-those-bearing-scars-ancient-disease/ (Accessed: 14 August 2020).

Sontag, S. (1989). *Aids and its Metaphors*. Toronto: Collins Publishers.

Wikipedia (n.d.). 'Social Distancing' [online]. Available at: https://en.wikipedia.org/wiki/Social_distancing (Accessed: 14 August 2020).

Notes

1. From the Greek λέπρα. The term translates the condition known as תערצ (sāraʿat) in the Pentateuch.
2. New English Translation, with some adjustments, e.g. here: תערצ = *lepra*.

Resilience in a Time of COVID-19 — Three Biblical Models

Plague, Uncleanness and Indigestion

Megan Warner

Introduction

It is perhaps timely that one of busiest fields of biblical criticism in recent years has been the employment of trauma theory as interpretive lens. Happily, biblical scholars have not been entirely unprepared for responding to COVID-19 with resources from within the tradition. Further, interest in the concept of 'resilience' as an offshoot of trauma theory has been growing, and I have been working in this field, as well as with trauma theory more generally, now for some years (Warner, 2020; Warner et al., 2020). In this trauma-focused work, scholars are mostly concerned with identifying how, and to what extent, the experience of trauma impacted upon biblical writing. Some, however, are concerned with how an awareness of the impact of trauma upon our Scriptures may help to inform public and pastoral theologians in adapting biblical models for application today.

In this paper I consider three possible biblical models from the Hebrew Bible (HB)): (i) the concept of divine plague, (ii) cultic regulations around uncleanness and isolation, and (iii) the presentation, within Priestly traditions, of the earth as an independent agent with a sensitive digestion system.

Biblical Resilience

There is no universally agreed definition of resilience, and academic literature about resilience as interpretive aid is still very limited. The definition that has won most support is that of the American Psychological Association, which describes resilience as 'the process of adapting well in the face of adversity, trauma, tragedy, threats or significant sources of stress ...' (American Psychological Association, 2012). The APA's page goes on to identify a range of 'factors' that will influence how much resilience a person demonstrates.

What does it mean for a piece of text to be resilient? Whitehead and Whitehead (2016) offer three resilience 'factors': 'relationship', 'reframing' and 'resolve'. One of these – reframing – is particularly relevant to assessing the resilience of literature. 'Reframing' is a technique of storytelling that harnesses the flexibility of the storyteller so that the story that an individual, or group, tells about itself (and by which it constructs its identity) can change or develop over time in response to experiences, good and bad, so as to permit the individual or group to prepare itself for the future.

William L. Randall, a gerontologist who writes about reframing and aging, argues that aging is a continuous process of setbacks, or minor traumas, and that an aging person needs to be flexible and to tell a 'good, strong story' about themselves if they are to remain resilient. He writes, 'A good strong story reaches out—in humility and awe—to something grander than ourselves, to a vaster narrative than that of our own little self, to [...] the "transcendent horizon of the life story"' (Randall, 2016, p. 9). Telling a story about ourselves that reaches out in this way, to something beyond ourselves, and that incorporates both the good and the bad, with a healthy dose of irony, is one of the best ways of building resilience.

The principal insight of trauma-informed biblical scholarship is that most of our biblical material was written during, or following, major experiences of trauma (Boase and Frechette, 2016). Given that our Scriptures have proven remarkably resilient – still shaping Western culture millennia later – they are also rich veins to be mined for techniques for reframing.

Divine Plague

Because we know something about the history of Ancient Israel, it is possible to trace biblical reframing, and to make informed guesses

Resilience in a Time of COVID-19 – Three Biblical Models

about how biblical theology and story-telling adapted in response to major calamity. 'Divine plague' has been, for most people, the first biblical imagery or model that has come to mind in the face of COVID-19. It is helpful to know something of the background to this imagery when thinking about COVID-19 because envisaging the virus as a divinely appointed plague has the potential to give rise to problematic theology.

Most of the plague stories from the HB can be dated either to the period of the exile itself, or to the period after the return. The plagues were reportedly sent for varying reasons. On some occasions the reason is the one that readers today most commonly associate with plagues – divine punishment, usually by YHWH against YHWH's own people, but sometimes by other gods or against other peoples. In other places, however, plagues are designed not as punishment, but as demonstrations of divine strength and power. This is so in the case of the Exodus plagues, for example (in P referred to as 'signs and wonders'). The long narrative of the plagues that preceded the departure of the Israelites from Egypt is an extended demonstration of the superiority of the strength and power of YHWH. YHWH is pitted against the magicians of Egypt, and wins at every stage, although because YHWH continues to harden the heart of Pharaoh, more and more dramatic displays of YHWH's power are called for.

Historical background can help us to understand the function of the model of divine plague. The destruction of Jerusalem in 587 BCE, and the removal of the top tiers of society to exile in Babylon, was an event that struck at the heart of the identity of Ancient Israel. Israel's God had previously travelled with her armies into battle, assuring them of victory even against forces of far greater numbers. What did it mean that YHWH's chosen people had been defeated in battle, and the Holy City and the Temple destroyed? The Israelites had a long time in exile to ponder this question.

There were many possible, albeit unpalatable, answers. Perhaps YHWH was not as strong as the Israelites had previously thought? Once they had been exposed to the people and gods of other nations in Babylonia, the Israelites had cause to wonder whether they had 'backed the right horse'. Even more disconcerting, had YHWH been strong all along, but fickle, and simply given up on the 'stiff-necked' Israelites? One answer, that avoided these unpalatable options, was that YHWH was neither weak nor fickle, but instead so strong as to be able to use foreign nations as agents to punish or deliver Israel. This was the answer that Israel chose, and which is demonstrated by the biblical accounts of divine plagues.

There are two principal reasons why the model of divine plague, however, would not serve us well, today, in the context of COVID-19. First, at least since the Holocaust it has been clear that a theology of divine punishment is unacceptable as a solution to the problem of theodicy in our world. The associated 'blaming' of the victim of a disaster is a stance that can no longer be maintained. Secondly, the use of the 'story' of divine punishment and displays of power did not, even in its original context, prove effective in the long term. 'Punishment' was a terrifically resilient model for those in exile in Babylon, yearning to return to the land of Canaan. Once the return had happened, however, it no longer worked as a resilient story. If divine punishment, plagues and exile would be the response to inevitable future failure to live up to YHWH's covenant standards, then how long could Israel maintain its covenant relationship, or survive an uncertain future in which further national defeats and exiles might become the norm?

Uncleanness and Isolation

The HB's accounts of leprosy offer us a potentially appealing model for consideration in relation to COVID-19. There is only a limited sense of leprosy as a divinely appointed punishment, and, crucially, there was a ritual process for effecting the cleansing of an unclean person or building. The cultic response was one of isolation of the leprous person – a kind of biblical social distancing, or shielding.

What is crucial in this approach is that the affected individual, rather than the community as a whole, is assigned responsibility for protecting the wider community. In its historical context this can be understood to have been a resilient development, meaning that the actions, or the health, of an individual could be sheeted home to that person rather than impacting the fate, and standing within the divine covenant, of Israel as a whole.

Despite the superficial parallels, however, the leprosy model has not been adopted internationally. It is a mark of our civility, I suggest, that immediate responses in the overwhelming majority of international settings have not placed the responsibility for the care of the community on the heads of infected individuals. Regretfully, then, I see little in the biblical model of management of leprous disease, that might be helpful in our own context, over and above an illustration of a process of resilient reframing that may in itself be instructive. For a far more detailed discussion of this biblical model see the essay by Justin Duff in this volume.

An earth with a weak digestive system

There appear to have been multiple Israelite reframing 'projects' going on in any one time, as different individuals or 'schools' put their own ideological or theological stamp on Israel's holy scriptures. One of the wonders of the HB is that texts produced as part of these disparate projects were not lost or supressed, but preserved alongside one another. The period following the return from Babylonian exile was especially generative. It is possible to identify two primary ideological/theological sets of responses to the experience of exile and the return. One, evidenced principally in Deuteronomy, Ezra and Nehemiah, had a national horizon, emphasising the need for strong identity boundaries and a return to an idealised Torah. The other, found in Priestly books such as Leviticus and Isaiah, had a universalistic horizon, finding a place and a role for Israel among the nations, and recognising YHWH as the creator of the whole earth.

It is in this latter, Priestly, outlook that I see a possible third model. In Priestly reframing the earth is presented not as an object, to be acted upon by human beings, but as an independent agent – sometimes with human characteristics, although of greater significance than human beings – capable of acting on its own volition.

The 'indigestion' referred to in the title is the earth's. The earth has its own vocation – to make a holy place, suitable for YHWH's home. To that end, the earth is punished by YHWH for its own defilement, and responds to the activities of people who defile it by vomiting them out (Lev 18:25, 28; 20:22). The earth functions as a self-cleansing mechanism. This is vastly different from the Deuteronomistic model of people and land. In D, either YHWH, or the people of Israel, or both together, have responsibility for driving non-Israelites out of the land that YHWH gives to Israel. In P, conversely, the land acts independently, and expels people according to their actions rather than their ethnicity.

The earth's digestive reflex system is not the only way in which it is acknowledged as an independent agent in P. In Leviticus 17-26 the punishment of *the land*, and not people, explains the destruction of Jerusalem and the Babylonian exile. The land, just as much as people, was required to keep the Sabbath (Lev 25:2), but the actions of people had prevented it from doing so. The long exile of the Israelites allowed the land to observe the sabbaths it had missed (Lev 26:43).

If the vocation of the land is to make an undefiled home for YHWH, what is the vocation of human beings? According to the creation narratives of Genesis 1-3, humans have two principal vocations. One is found in Gen 1:28, 'God blessed them, and God said to them, "Be fruitful and multiply", ...'. The other is found in Genesis 2. The 'second' account of creation, that begins in Gen 2:4b, opens with a focus on the earth, and the fact that it had not yet become fruitful because YHWH Elohim had not yet caused rain to fall or provided anyone to serve it (Gen 2:5). This is the tension that drives the ensuing narrative. YHWH Elohim responds in two ways, first appointing rivers to water the land and then making an *adam* (literally an 'earth creature') from the dust of the earth (*adamah*) (Gen 2:7), and putting the *adam* in a garden to serve and watch/keep the *Adamah* (Gen 2:15). When YHWH Elohim observes that it isn't good for the *adam* to be alone, a quest to find a helper for the *adam* is launched. The effect of all this (although we humans have often been too focused on the relationship between the man and the woman to notice) is to make the wellbeing of the earth primary, with humans a secondary creation designed to serve and service the earth. We have tended to read anthropocentrically, privileging the vocation to subdue and have dominion over the earth over that to serve it.

The model I am suggesting is one in which the earth itself is responsible for having generated the virus. Without necessarily wanting to pick up every nuance of the Priestly model, I do want to suggest that to conceptualise COVID-19 as an expression of the earth's self-care may be a resilient exercise in reframing. The consequences of the virus, from the earth's point of view, have been a reduction (albeit limited) in human population and a dramatic reduction, even almost a cessation, of the most damaging elements of human contribution to climate change – travel (particularly air travel) and industrial production and pollution. We all know that these activities will return, but one of the resilient benefits of understanding the pandemic as planetary self-care may be the recognition that change to the way we relate to the earth is necessary and urgent, and that failure to heed this warning will inevitably lead to more, and more extreme, disruption of our lifestyles. Are there other resilience benefits?

The model may help human beings to build a more realistic picture of our place in the created order – first God, then the earth and then humans. It could build a connection between our experience of the virus and our role and responsibility to our environment. It would grant agency to human beings, one of the things that people most need if they are to avoid becoming 'stuck' in trauma response. In terms of Randall's concept of the 'good strong story', this model places our recent experience in the context of a broader, cosmic, story. It helps to define a positive identity for human beings – loved children of God, entrusted with care of God's good creation and with responsibility for, as well as influence upon, how creation treats us.

This is not a perfect model, certainly. It still incorporates a concept of divine punishment (*which should not be over-emphasised*), and leaves open questions of equity between nations, already grappling with patterns of climate change in which the actions of the developed West impact disproportionately those nations with the fewest resources. Nevertheless, I hope that I have managed to demonstrate the potential for it to be a resilient and regenerative model.

Conclusions

This paper has set out to do two principal things. First, to highlight the importance of the reframing of identity stories, and to point to the resilience of the biblical writings in this regard. Secondly, it considers some reframing options in the text of our experience of COVID-19. The third model, emphasising the agency of the earth, is the supported option – bringing together long-held, biblical, imagery of loving creator, loved creation and (only then) trusted, responsible creatures. This is not one of the best-known and appreciated biblical models, but perhaps it deserves to be.

Dr Megan Warner is Tutor in Old Testament, Northern College, Luther King House, Manchester.

Questions for Discussion

1. Does this model have an *affective* impact on you?

2. How important is it for Christians to frame (or 'reframe') natural events in biblical language, imagery or models, if at all?

3. Is resilience a wholly positive thing in your view?

References

American Psychological Association (2012). 'Building Your Resilience' [online]. Available at: www.APA.org/topics/resilience (Accessed: 28 July 2020).

Boase, E. and Frechette, C. G. (eds.) (2016). *Bible Through the Lens of Trauma*. Atlanta: SBL.

Randall, W. L. (2013). 'The importance of Being Ironic: Narrative Openness and Personal Resilience in Later Life', *The Gerontologist*, 53, pp. 9-16.

Warner, M. (2020). *Joseph: A story of resilience*. London: SPCK.

Warner, M. et al. (eds.) (2020). *Tragedies and Christian Congregations: The Practical Theology of Trauma*. London/New York: Routledge.

Whitehead, J. D. and Whitehead, E. E. (2016). *The Virtue of Resilience*. Maryknoll, NY: Orbis.

Paschal Simultaneity in Time of Pandemic

A Liturgical Theological Response to COVID-19

Ann Swailes

A connection is often posited between particularly intense and extensive exposure to suffering and especially incisive and energetic exploration of its theological significance. It is possible to identify a series of historical contexts in which especially concentrated, and distinctive, doctrinal, homiletic and devotional attention has been given to the theology of suffering. The Lisbon earthquake of November 1st, 1755, whose death toll was swollen by the numbers of worshippers trapped inside the city's churches which collapsed in the course of All Saints' Day Mass; the wholesale slaughter of the First World War and especially both the genocidal atrocities and use of atomic weapons in the course of the Second, are all regularly cited as examples. In face of COVID-19, it seems we are currently living through one such cultural moment. It is thus helpful to consider what can be learned through dialogue with inhabitants of previous ages whose theological sensibility was contoured equally deeply by suffering.

Accordingly I shall ask, in conversation with Julian of Norwich and William Langland, how texts drawn from Late Medieval England (another era, as various dubiously tasteful memes currently doing the rounds of the internet put it, of two popes and a pandemic) might energise and inspire contemporary theology of suffering. In particular, I suggest that their writings provide evidence of what might be called an aesthetic of paschal simultaneity, with important implications for pastoral practice today. What I mean by 'paschal simultaneity' is that the juxtapositions of Christ's dying and rising in each text enables the light of Easter glory to illuminate the anguish of Good Friday. This orients those who suffer towards a horizon of hope, while celebration of the Resurrection is preserved from triumphalist insensitivity to suffering by recollection of the Cross.

I shall approach these Medieval witnesses indirectly, via two contrasting approaches to the mystery of suffering which both loomed large in the theological landscape of late modernity. The first is the doctrine of divine passibility, which holds that God suffers, not only in the context of the Incarnation, but eternally in the divine nature itself, thus providing human sufferers with an inexhaustible source of empathetic comprehension. The second is incorporationist ecclesiology, which stresses how baptism engrafts human beings into Christ's body the Church. Thus the suffering of Christians becomes not merely an imitation of, but a genuine participation in the saving passion of Christ. On this account, such suffering has an objective utility, which endows its bearers with subjective dignity.

Passibilist doctrines of God and incorporationist ecclesiologies, respectively unthinkable and axiomatic for Julian and Langland, can thus be considered as competing responses to human pain. In what follows, using resources drawn from liturgical theology, I shall suggest that the more ecclesially focused approach contains more promising resources for the chastening of the pathological attraction to distress which – paradoxically – both risk legitimizing.

I am aware that this preference is not only, for many, counter-intuitive. It is also dependent on a perspective which may seem currently especially vulnerable.

Incorporationist ecclesiology makes it possible to speak of liturgy analogically as both the Church's official worship and the lived experience of Christians. If liturgy is defined etymologically as work on behalf of the people, then, on the incorporationist account, Christ is the liturgist par excellence. He is the one whose saving work is set forth and rendered available in the Church's worship, but who also continues this work in the actions and passions of Christians and Christian communities, who constitute the body of which Christ is the head.

This radical identification of head and members bestows on the suffering of Christians its derivative redemptive significance, giving incorporationist ecclesiology its distinctive consolatory potential. However, the consequences of COVID-19 for current ecclesial praxis pose an acute pastoral challenge here. How are we to see the relationship between churchly and mundane liturgy, when access to worship in church is restricted or even impossible? The physical, mental and spiritual suffering occasioned by the pandemic simultaneously provides abundant occasion to reflect on how Christian suffering mirrors and participates in that of Christ, and requires that we have something consolatory to say to those who suffer. But to use the language of *liturgy* to express such consolation, when in the most obvious sense liturgical participation is in abeyance, is to risk speaking with profoundly damaging insensitivity. Nevertheless, because it is specifically a *paschal* incorporationist ecclesiology in which I seek to root a response to the mystery of suffering, I suggest there may prove grounds for hope even within the prolonged Good Friday so many are still experiencing after the end of Eastertide. The pastoral challenge might thus also be conceived as an opportunity.

Divine passibility was widely canvassed in the mid to late twentieth century as a new orthodoxy, the sole doctrine of God that could command intellectual and ethical respect in the light of the sufferings of the age. But recent evidence suggests that earlier reports of the demise of the theological impassibilism, which held sway for the majority of Christian history, have been somewhat exaggerated. This is not least because of concern about the potential weakening of ethical and political nerve implicit in theological passibilism. If, after all, God suffers, then it is perhaps neither possible, nor desirable, to work strenuously to overcome suffering in the creatures made in the divine image.

Meanwhile, although the radical repercussions of the twentieth century's large scale violent socio-political turmoil on theology are undeniable, it is clearly equally untenable to view Christian reflection on suffering as a late modern innovation. If our forebears responded to war, famine and indeed pandemic and societal upheaval in different, though equally sophisticated theological terms, resources from older approaches may perhaps be liberated for contemporary consolatory service.

If incorporationist ecclesiology is to fulfil this role, however, it too needs to be comprehensively purged of its own tendency to bestow a spurious glamour on human suffering. On this account, the sufferings of the faithful are derivatively but really the sufferings of Christ, and thus help forward nothing less than the redemption of the world. In consequence, that exacerbation of suffering by the sense of absurdity that so often accompanies it is avoided, or at least mitigated, but it might well seem that consolation is here bought at too high a cost. It is a disturbingly short step, after all, from saying that suffering has some kind of objective, redemptive value, to saying that the more one suffers the better, and it is a step that has not infrequently been taken in the history of Christian spirituality, sometimes with catastrophic consequence.

It is here that the insights of liturgical theology come into play. If the imitation of Christ is viewed more or less exclusively as the imitation of his Passion, there is an obvious temptation to pathological dalliance with distress. If, however, one's gaze is synoptically fixed on Good Friday and Easter Sunday, participation in Christ's sufferings becomes *simultaneously* participation in his resurrection, so providing hope for an eschatological future free of pain and preventing an unhealthy exaltation of suffering as an end in itself.

Such synopsis is presupposed in classic Catholic theology of the liturgy. The Mass, after all, is simultaneously the sacred banquet as pledge of future glory and the renewed memorial of Christ's Passion, the re-presentation of Calvary. Insofar as the liturgy of the sanctuary resembles the liturgy of Christian life, something similar must be said of the way in which Christian pain finds itself immersed in Christ's Passion. The sufferings of Christians may partake of the saving value of the sufferings of Christ, but that value is itself dependent on the resurrection, without which Calvary would be simply the scene of judicial murder. The resurrection is not, however, merely the undoing of the Crucifixion, as though the Passion was somehow an absurd mistake. Rather, Cross and Resurrection are mutually interpretative. There is thus a kind of coincidence between the successive episodes of the story of Holy Week: as scripture, and liturgical, devotional and indeed artistic tradition all attest, Christ reigns from the Cross, but rises with his scars.

Granted this general principle of paschal simultaneity, it is clearly possible either to view Good Friday through the lens of Easter, or vice versa, perspectives that might be called 'retrojective' and 'projective' respectively. The retrojective form of paschal simultaneity, validated by the Johannine account of the first Holy Week, and echoed in the evocations of the ritual of martial triumph that becomes a commonplace in Patristic preaching on the Passion is historically predominant. After all, the consolatory potential in seeing one's sufferings as already suffused with resurrection light is evident. This is exemplifed in churchly liturgy in the Alleluias of the Byzantine Good Friday burial of Christ, for instance. But it is also manifest in the luminosity of many artistic, musical and poetic evocations of the

Passion, from the bejewelled though bloody Cross of the Old English *Dream of the Rood*, through the radiant backdrop of Fra Angelico's San Marco crucifixion frescoes to the final numbers of the St Matthew Passion. This allows for the possibility of discerning Christ-like beauty not in suffering per se, but in its being borne co-compassionately by members of Christ's body. Thus the mundane liturgy of Christian life reflects the sufferings of Christ sacramentally enacted in the liturgy of the sanctuary.

There is perhaps less immediately evident appeal in the complementary, projective, approach whereby Easter is viewed in the light of Good Friday. Arguably, it is to be found, in, for instance, the Medieval practice of reprising the Good Friday veneration of the Cross on Easter morning, but there are undoubtedly fewer texts and artefacts in which this perspective is unambiguously present. This too is predictable: amnesia, personal and communal, in the face of suffering is a widely recognised – and readily comprehensible – phenomenon. However, it is perhaps precisely this version of paschal simultaneity that is particularly needed today.

If both passibilist theology and incorporationist ecclesiology require redemption from an unhealthy exaltation of suffering, there is a more subtle pathology to which an exclusively retrojective perspective on paschal simultaneity is potentially prey. While both passibilist doctrines of God and an incompletely paschal ecclesiology of the Mystical Body threaten to foreshorten the Holy Triduum by halting at Good Friday, an exclusively retrojective simultaneity threatens to prioritise Easter Sunday equally unilaterally. Here the Crucifixion comes to be regarded potentially as simply a reversible misfortune, a downward blip on an otherwise uninterrupted upward trajectory, with the attendant risk of evacuating Christ's suffering, and derivatively that of Christians, of much of its meaning. A complementary backward glance from Garden to Cross might provide a suggestive corrective.

It is frequently noted that the notion of suffering as something simply to be annihilated, with the consequently disabling sense of anomaly where this proves impossible, forms part of a distinctively modern sensibility. It is one perhaps particularly called in question by our current experience of pandemic. Later Medieval responses to trauma and sorrow, in particular, are rarely either so ambitious, or, (perhaps in consequence), so unambiguously negative. It is here in particular that I suggest Julian of Norwich and William Langland may reinvigorate our contemporary discourse.

Julian and Langland both portray the abiding scars of crucifixion on the body of the risen Lord, and the wounds to which they provide a point of entry, as making a significant contribution to an incorporationist ecclesiology which is neither pathologically fixated on suffering nor evasively focused on its impermanence.

Julian's evocation of the *feyer and delectable place* (Glasscoe, 1993, p. 35) reached through the wound in the side of Jesus, large enough to provide shelter for all those who will be saved, emphasises not only the savingly hospitable, but in consequence also the ecclesiologically fruitful nature of Christ's scars. If the wounds of Christ are redemptive, this is because they open up his body, allowing access which is simultaneously incorporation in the most literal sense, with all that this implies about the identity and dignity of the Christian suffering subject. Julian finds no difficulty in accepting the paradox of a now impassible Christ continually suffering in his members. She neither amplifies this paradox systematically nor draws the conclusions later Catholic spirituality will do for devotional praxis, but there is nonetheless perhaps potential here for such development.

Langland's evocation of the abiding fissures in Christ's resurrection body functions ultimately in the same ecclesiological interests. Passus XVIII of the B-text of *Piers Plowman* forms the dramatic climax of the poem in which Langland's narrator, Will, falls asleep during the paraliturgical preliminaries to Palm Sunday Mass, and finds himself present in dream at the Crucifixion and Christ's post mortem descent into hell. Immediately after the Harrowing of Hell, simultaneously the moment of Christ's deepest abasement and highest exaltation, the dreamer is roused from sleep by the bells calling him to his Easter duties, and stays awake long enough to get to Mass with his wife and daughter, and be present as far as the offertory, before slumbering again.

Highly significantly, the opening of the dream that follows has a figure appear 'paynted al blody/and come in with a Crosse bifor the commune peple'. The figure is 'right lyke in alle lymes to oure Lorde Jhesu', and, indeed, Conscience confirms that, though he is dressed in Piers' heraldic colours, this is, indeed 'Cryst with his Crosse'. Easter then shades into Pentecost, conceived in strikingly ecclesiological terms. There is a brief allusion to the account of Acts 2 before the scene shifts to a meticulously allegorical construction, of a house formed of Christ's sufferings, with scripture for its roof and a cement called 'mercy' concocted from Christ's 'baptismal blood'. The house is to be called 'Unity', glossed as a proper ecclesiological name ('holy Church in English'). It is thus unavoidably stressed that the communion which characterises the Church as the Mystical Body is inextricably founded in the abidingly fruitful wounds of Christ.

'Unitee' is almost immediately attacked by a combination of natural disaster and human sin, causing devastation so great that Conscience, upon whom the narrative spotlight is now fixed, leaves in order to seek Piers Plowman, 'the only one who can put down pride', elsewhere (Robertson and Shepherd, 2006, p. 333).

It is perhaps precisely here where the poem's centre of consolatory gravity is, however counter-intuitively, to be located. Strikingly, it is also where its projective paschal simultaneity is most potent. The Passion of Christ needs must be performed in the life of a Church whose bodily unity with Christ is grounded in his Eucharistic body. But it also partakes fully of contingency and frailty, as did indeed the body of the historical Jesus, despite the consubstantial unity of his humanity with impassible divinity. There is therefore no route by which pilgrimage in search of truth, or of Piers the Plowman, will ultimately reach its goal, except through imitative participation in the Passion, Harrowing of Hell, Resurrection and Ascension.

The ambiguous perceptions of the resurrected body in each author witness neither to a pathological exaltation of Good Friday at the expense of Easter, then, nor to an Easter that erases memory of the preceding days of the Triduum, but to a therapeutic simultaneity in the life of believer and believing community alike.

Both authors, consequently, provoke the question: how might Christian response to the mystery of suffering today be enriched by more conscious reflection on paschal simultaneity? And what difference might it make to our liturgy and to our preaching, churchly and mundane?

Sr Ann Swailes, OP is a member of the English Dominican Congregation of St Catherine of Siena, a doctoral candidate at Clare College, Cambridge, and assistant Roman Catholic Chaplain to the University of Cambridge.

Questions for Discussion

1. Is it possible to speak responsibly of Christ-like beauty in the bearing of suffering, and what contribution might this make to theological reflection on human pain?

2. In the light of the current pandemic, how can we live as 'Christ the liturgist' in the world, in virtue of our membership of his Body the Church, when we are unable to attend to Christ as liturgist in the sanctuary?

References

Glasscoe, M. (ed.) (1993). *Julian of Norwich: A Revelation of Love.* Exeter: Exeter University Press.

Robertson, E. and Shepherd, S. H. A. (eds.) (2006). *William Langland, Piers Plowman.* New York: Norton and Company.

A Theological Engagement with T. S. Eliot's The Waste Land

in the Context of COVID-19

Andrew Picard and Jaimee van Gemerden

The declarative opening line of T. S. Eliot's *The Waste Land* is that 'April is the cruellest month'. It is cruel because the hope of spring and new life clashes with the realities of suffering in the undead city. As COVID-19 escalated, April was, once again, perceived by some as the cruellest month. As Holy Week approached, U.S. Surgeon General Dr. Jerome Adams warned Americans to brace for the hardest and saddest week of their lives (Law, 2020). Whatever the merits of this assessment, the coincidence with Holy Week invites theological reflections on suffering and hope. This paper draws *The Waste Land* into conversation with the work of Donald MacKinnon and Karen Kilby to explore Christian accounts of suffering and hope amidst COVID-19. Eliot's poem is especially poignant as it arises in the post-war and post-pandemic context of the Spanish Flu outbreak in 1918-19, which Eliot and Vivien, his wife, contracted. Elizabeth Outka argues that the pandemic setting of the poem is often overlooked: 'despite the wealth of readings, critics have missed the poem's viral context' (Outka, 2020, 143). A pandemic reading does not supplant other interpretations, but further textures the richness of the poem, and offers insights into human experience amidst the trauma of war and a viral epidemic that open horizons for theological reflections on suffering and hope in COVID-19.

Theology and the tragedy of COVID-19's waste land

Residents of the waste land experience living death, an existential state where life and death exist simultaneously due to the meaninglessness of their situation. The first section of the poem, 'The Burial of the Dead', raises the idea of the allure of death and the zombie-like state of the characters' lives. The vision of human experience that Eliot's poem captures highlights the consequences of an absence of meaning in life, and the function of death in relation to meaning loss and meaning creation. Such an existential state resonates with some experiences amidst the global consequences of COVID-19 and the tragedy inherent in a pandemic context.

The relation of tragedy and theology is complex; Donald MacKinnon utilizes the literary category of tragedy to stress the need for theological realism, and an account of Christ's historical life in all its tragic dimensions (MacKinnon, 1968, 100). Some affirmations of Christ as victor suffer too much from superficial cosmic optimism, which reduces Easter to little more than a 'simple whoop of triumph' (MacKinnon, 1987, 200). The agony and tragedy of the cross are vanquished in the blinding light of the resurrection that assumes the world, which knows the extremities of pandemics, can be consoled by 'a remote metaphysical chatter' (MacKinnon, 1968, 92). Such easy resolutions fool theologians into believing they have reached solutions for suffering and evil when in fact they have barely begun to articulate the problems. Instead of providing an abstract resolution to evil, MacKinnon argues that the contradictions of Jesus's tragic history be given much greater prominence. There is a resolutely tragic element to the Christian faith, and MacKinnon refuses to leave unplumbed the depths of human grief inherent in Christ's life and death. The obedient life that is raised from the dead leads from the highways of success 'to the narrow defiles of failure and bewilderment' (MacKinnon, 2011, 256). Tragedy is not, in MacKinnon's assessment, the antithesis of hope, but a fundamental aspect of its gospel basis. Resurrection faith plunges the church into life within history, and all its tragedy, and requires we accept the burden of our humanity and solidarity with fellow humans (MacKinnon, 2011, 260).

MacKinnon's emphasis on the place of tragedy provides a perspective from which to encounter the human experience of suffering that Eliot explores in his poem. In the final stanzas of 'The Burial of the Dead', Eliot outlines his daily commute to the financial district, which is juxtaposed with allusions to Dante's *Inferno*, and the speaker states, 'a crowd flowed over London Bridge, so many' (line 62). The poet continues, quoting the third Canto of the Inferno which describes the observation of the dead on the banks of the Acheron; the crowds are ambiguous, neither inside of Hell nor out of it. The Thames becomes Eliot's Acheron, London his hell, and the crowd of commuters those who are 'undone' by death but still live their day to day existence in London. The residents of Eliot's London endure a state of life without meaningful existence due to their experience of tragedy. The suffering in Eliot's poem is so tragic that there can be no meaning conceived of within human existence. It is an extent of suffering that demands a vision of hope amidst, not in spite of, tragedy. Eliot's exposition of suffering accords with MacKinnon's demand that any account of hope that does not go through the narrow gate of suffering offers meaningless hope because it is abstracted from the bracing realities of life. The human experience of suffering cannot be lost within Christian accounts of hope that deny the experience of the sort of tragedy that Eliot's text highlights. Yet, such a claim requires careful theological nuance.

The theological limits of suffering and hope

The relation of suffering and hope in theology is complex, and Karen Kilby's apophaticism delineates some necessary theological limits. There are dual issues of intelligibility when it comes to a theological examination of suffering and hope. In relation to the mystery of suffering, there is a lack of intelligibility, and in relation to the mystery of God, there is an excess of intelligibility. These are not two sides of one coin, but a double apophatic pressure that acknowledges our inability to speak or theologise in the face of the mystery of God *and* the mystery of suffering (Kilby, 2017, 291). Given the lack of intelligibility about suffering Kilby helpfully stresses the need for something like apophaticism regarding theological accounts of suffering.

Western culture is excessively fearful of suffering, vulnerability, and limitation, and tends to deem suffering as a mark of failure. Rightly, theologians offer correctives to such tendencies, but there is a risk of going too far. The acceptance of suffering is often conflated with the embrace of suffering and celebration of vulnerability as determinative of not only human being but also divine being. The drive to say something meaningful about suffering often results in theodicies that assert a passible God who cannot be blamed for suffering because God is the one who suffers the most (Kilby, 2003, 21). Such approaches seek to reconcile God with suffering as the one whose eternal being is conditioned by suffering, but in doing so diminish the scandal of meaningless suffering. We persuade ourselves 'that suffering is not, in the end, when you come down to it, if you can look at it in just the right way, so very bad after all' (Kilby, 2019, 13). These claims are too knowing about the mystery of suffering and the mystery of God's ineffable being. In place of such knowingness about suffering, Kilby (2020, 174) suggests a restraint of speech and knowledge that resists making meaning where meaning may not exist, or we have no right to ascribe it. Given the horrific impacts of COVID-19, there is a need for a more restrained theology that respects the lack of intelligibility regarding the virus's traumatic effects on patients, families, medical workers, economies, and global politics. There is a proper limit to what theology can claim in the face of suffering, and some forms of meaningless suffering are not able to be resituated into a story that gives us comfort (Kilby, 2019, 7).

What is lacking in many theological engagements with suffering 'is any sense of bafflement before suffering, of being silenced by it, brought to the end of what can be explained' (Kilby, 2019, 4). There is a failure of language and knowledge when faced with meaningless suffering; our explanatory methods are silenced. A greater restraint in Christian eschatology means that Christian visions of hope cannot be applied to every situation to derive consolation. We cannot fill out the detail of eschatological hope without risking further pain and suffering from our meaning-making. Whilst we may hope that suffering is woven into something meaningful and redemptive, 'we cannot even begin to imagine what that might be, to conceive of what could make meaningful, or understandable, or acceptable, the terrors that befall other people' (Kilby, 2017, 291). Kilby's apophatic tension in eschatology resonates with the inherent tensions raised by the representation of the loss of meaning in *The Waste Land*.

In Eliot's *The Waste Land*, there is a desire for illumination, but revelation and meaning are impotent. The lack of the stabilizing force of a central figure in the poem gives way to a polyphony of perspectives that search for revelation which is found to be unintelligible in the wake of such suffering. The voices of the poem's prophets, the Sibyl, Madame Sosostris, and Tiresias, interweave with the lives of the waste land's inhabitants offering only riddles and silence in response to their questions. In a fragmented world, the knowledge of the seers is meaningless and just as incapable of expressing reality as any other visionary voice. The seemingly minor character of the ancient seer Tiresias unifies the many prophetic voices that speak in an attempt to create meaning in a context where it is sought but remains elusive. Tiresias is a symbol of prophetic impotence who sees but cannot communicate his knowledge with characters for whom suffering has made meaningful revelation nonsensical. Eliot's prophetic characters exemplify Kilby's stress upon the unintelligibility of suffering. Accounts of Christian eschatology need to uphold the unintelligibility of meaningless suffering in tension with hope.

The place of suffering within Christian eschatological accounts

Christian eschatology, Kilby (2003, 24-25) suggests, must uphold three features of theology, all of which are desirable, but not all of which are achievable. Eschatology ought to 'provide a fully Christian picture of God; it ought to give, or at least leave room for, a full recognition of the injustice, terror and tragedy we participate in and see around us; and it ought to be coherent' (Kilby, 2003, 25). Yet, not all of these three can be achieved and sacrifices must be made. Whilst theodicies often sacrifice a full recognition of evil or a fully Christian picture of God to maintain coherence, Kilby sacrifices the possibility of a fully coherent theological vision in the light of the mystery of divine being and the mystery of suffering. However, does Kilby's necessary emphasis upon the lack of knowing drive out some of the positive claims that may be made? In Christian eschatology there is continuity and discontinuity; there is divine hiddenness *and* divine revealedness; the New Jerusalem is like and unlike Eden; the risen Christ is recognizable and unrecognizable; and the post-resurrection disciples are knowing and unknowing. What can be said theologically about suffering and hope without committing the moral transgression of excessive knowingness?

The eschatological tension within accounts of suffering and hope leads to the ultimate question of Eliot's poem: is there the possibility for renewed life or is death the ideal release? The ending of 'What the Thunder Said' leads some scholars to believe it outlines a vision of hope for restoration in the future, while others claim that there is no redemption for the waste land.[1] The final stanza of *The Waste Land* opens with the voice of the Fisher King whose desire for personal regeneration and the restoration of the land is explicit in the way that his act of fishing suggests waiting for the appearance of the 'Divine Life symbol' (Weston, 1920, 127). As Eliot's character fishes at the end of the poem the question of regeneration remains at the forefront of the text. Can life be restored in the waste land or should the king 'set [his] lands in order' to anticipate death? The Fisher King asks himself this question as the state of the poem changes into disconnected fragments that culminate in the meditative repetition of the Sanskrit word 'Shantih'. Shantih, which Eliot translates as 'the Peace which passeth understanding', is traditionally understood as a 'verse invocation seeking the blessings of gods and sages in one's pursuit of spiritual wisdom' (Chandran 1989: 682). Rather than being understood as a statement of peace, K. Narayana Chandran (1989: 683) argues that '"shantih" here is not so much wished as wished for'. Eliot's use of 'shantih' forms a benediction that alludes to the desire for peace in the place of a hope for restoration, a desire that is left unfulfilled by the final lines of the poem.

The hope for restoration sits in tension with the experience of suffering in *The Waste Land* and COVID-19, and needs to remain a tension. Can anything be said theologically in this tension without committing moral transgressions regarding the suffering of others (Kilby 2017, 289)? Whilst we cannot pretend to offer a fully coherent theology of suffering and hope, the biblical witness offers hints and suggestions that constrain a flat apophaticism, and opens possibilities for knowing within unknowingness. MacKinnon maintains that the scars and wounds of the risen Christ invite us to see continuity between Christ's suffering and his resurrected life (MacKinnon, 1968, 95). Likewise, Kilby considers the significance of the wounds in the resurrected body of Christ, and notes that they offer a way of thinking about hope that is not mere forgetfulness of what has gone before (Kilby, 2017, 290). Post-resurrection, Christ's scars are not dispensed with, and they are revelatory to Thomas and the disciples. The resurrection, MacKinnon argues, is not a dramatic Hollywood reversal narrative, but the vindication of Christ's faithful life in and through suffering (MacKinnon, 1968, 95). This need not lead to the knowing assertions of Christian hope that Kilby cautions against. Instead, it follows the traces of scripture that suggest human suffering is vindicated, not vanquished, and remembered, not forgotten, in the one through whom all things cohere (MacKinnon, 1968, 96). We cannot offer robust assertions of meaning regarding suffering in COVID-19, but we are invited to see that Christian hope is found in Christ's presence in and through suffering, and not aside from it.

Jaimee van Gemerden is a Graduate Student in Theology, Carey Graduate School, Carey Baptist College, New Zealand.

Andrew Picard is Director of Carey Graduate School and Lecturer in Theology and Culture, Carey Baptist College, New Zealand.

Questions for Discussion

1. In what ways does a recognition of the tragedy and unknowability of suffering contribute to a more fruitful response to the experience of COVID-19?

2. How can the image of the scars borne by the risen Christ signal a new form of Christian hope?

References

Chandran, K. N., 1989, '"Shantih" in *The Waste Land*', *American Literature*, 61 (4), pp. 681-683.

Eliot, T. S., 1971, *The Waste Land: A Facsimile and Transcript of the Original Drafts including the Annotations of Ezra Pound*, Eliot V. (ed.), London: Faber and Faber.

Kilby, K., 2003, 'Evil and the Limits of Theology', *New Blackfriars* 84 (983), pp. 13-29.

Kilby, K., 2017, 'Eschatology, Suffering and the Limits of Theology', in Chalame, C. et al (eds.), *Game Over? Reconsidering Eschatology*, Berlin, De Gruyter, pp. 279-91.

Kilby, K., 2019, 'Negative Theology and Meaningless Suffering', *Modern Theology* 36 (1), pp. 92-104.

Kilby, K., 2020, 'The Seductions of Kenosis', in Davies, R. and Kilby, K. (eds.), *Suffering and the Christian Life*, London: T&T Clark, pp. 163-74.

Knapp Hay, E., 2014, *T. S. Eliot's Negative Way*, Cambridge: Harvard University Press.

Law, T., 2020, 'Surgeon General Adams Warns of "Saddest Week of

Most Americans' Lives" as COVID-19 Pandemic Spreads', *Time*, 6 April [online]. Available at: https://time.com/5815870/jerome-adams-surgeon-general-saddest-week-covid-19/ (Accessed 19 May 2020).

MacKinnon, D. M., 1968, *Borderlands of Theology, and Other Essays by Donald M. MacKinnon*, Roberts, G. W. and Smucker, D. E. (eds.), London: Lutterworth Press.

MacKinnon, D. M., 2011, 'The Tomb was Empty', in McDowell, J. (ed) *Philosophy and the Burden of Theological Honesty: A Donald MacKinnon Reader*, London: T&T Clark, pp. 255-260.

MacKinnon, D. M., 1987, *Themes in Theology: The Three-fold Chord; Essays in Philosophy, Politics and Theology*, Edinburgh: T&T Clark.

Outka, E., 2020, *Viral Modernism: The Influenza Pandemic and Interwar Literature*, Columbia: Columbia University Press.

Weston, J., 1920, *From Ritual to Romance*, Reprint, Garden City: Anchor Books, 1957.

Notes

1. Eloise Knapp Hay argues that the focus of the poem 'is not toward the Fisher King's desire for renewed life but toward hope for cessation of this cycle of rebirths' (Knapp Hay, 2014, 54).

Virtual Communion, COVID-19, and the Nature of the Body of Christ

Hannah Bowman and Neil Dhingra

Introduction

In his memoirs, Jürgen Moltmann (2009) describes two different Eucharists in which he participated in 1968. One was with Protestants and Catholics at the London offices of the publisher Sheed and Ward before an anti-Vietnam War protest. The second was at the historic St Giles Cathedral in Edinburgh, after a formal lecture, where the Lord's Supper was served on silver trays by uniformed servers. To Moltmann, the first celebration evoked Christ's presence; the second left him depressed. Of course, the first Eucharist challenged denominational boundaries and connected him to the 'streets of the poor who follow Jesus', but Moltmann also distinguishes the two Eucharists in physical language. At the first, 'Bread and wine passed from hand to hand in a small circle'; at the second, 'The participants sat separate from one another, scattered here and there in the great church' (Moltmann, 2009, p. 164).

How does physical presence matter? In this essay, we explore the possibility of a 'virtual Eucharist' using Moltmann's theology of God's suffering. We ask whether the sense of Christ's presence is bound up with a congregation and material signs that are not merely inclusive but physically present—like on the floor of a Catholic publisher in London—or whether the nature of the Eucharist derives from a sense of absence that reflects the absence of God to the crucified Jesus. This essay originated in a blog post by Hannah Bowman (Bowman, 2020). Neil Dhingra responded in the comments; correspondence began. We disagree about Moltmann's theology, and therefore about the possibility or indeed desirability of a 'virtual Eucharist', but we agree that the question of the 'virtual Eucharist' should be less about technological ingenuity and more about the nature of God.

The debate over virtual communion

During this pandemic, C. Andrew Doyle (2020), Bishop of the Episcopal Diocese of Texas, issued a pastoral letter arguing against celebrations of virtual communion because of the necessity of a physical congregation. To Doyle, worship must be a self-consciously communal activity in 'one place' with 'physical material signs.' A virtual Eucharist risks being an 'abstraction' celebrated by a community that can only be a 'precursor' to those gathered 'shoulder to shoulder and hand in hand'. Uniquely, a physical gathering is the experience of a 'transcendent reality' that transforms as 'eyes, hearts, and minds are lifted up in a different way to hear and see differently'—an experience unavailable to individuals linked online (see McGowan, 2020).

Doyle's concern that virtual communion remains an expression of individual preferences, however deeply felt, echoes Graham Ward's concerns that cyberspace, with its fluid realities and infinite possibilities, is just individual desire writ large (Ward, 2000). On the other hand, supporters of virtual communion have argued that being online is neither lesser than nor different from physical presence, at least as far as internal states go. Virtual *and* physical reality seem capable of bearing 'an orientation of the heart and soul' (Stoddard, 2020). One can be mentally or spiritually absent in both settings, and sincere or insincere with and without a computer.

Others see the distinction itself as outdated. 'A young mother wrestles her toddler into a shopping cart with one hand and updates her Facebook status with her other' (Reklis, 2012), present seamlessly throughout. One might be physically there at a church service but listen through digital sound. Virtual environments may be fully immersive; physical environments can involve partial sensibility (Rundell, 2019). Our virtual world seems neither extraneous to nor a pale facsimile of brick-and-mortar 'real life'.

Virtual communion and remote distance education

Is there, then, a specific desire evoked by physical presence? Doyle's argument for 'transcendent reality' resembles the late philosopher Hubert Dreyfus' argument for in-person teaching. In Dreyfus' phenomenological interpretation (2009), a classroom has a shared mood to which we become attuned with our body's movements. The shared context, equivalent to the 'depth of field' for a football player, lets students be more involved in the class (and the teacher to be more effective) (Dreyfus, 2009, p. 66). This mood is not confected by individual desires, but created by a focal practice that provides a background, a self-contained world in which gestures and movements allow for the sense of shared communion that makes for an exciting class, or, Dreyfus acknowledges, the sacredness in Seder or a (non-virtual) Eucharist. When Doyle (2020) says of the physical Eucharist, 'We are different when we are together', and speaks of an 'awakening' and something we 'come to understand', he implicitly refers to the sense of attunement: 'We cannot have a feast of friends alone.' This attunement shapes, as Graham Ward (2000) may say, the distinctive desire evoked by the communion of the church.

The pandemic has not only seen arguments for and against virtual communion but has required widespread remote distance education. Its shortcomings seem to confirm Dreyfus' arguments. As Mark Vernon (2020) has written, in online environments we cannot *feel* what others mean but must prioritize one of our senses and actively try to capture our conversation partners' meanings. Online meetings are also inhospitable to the subtleties of movement and gesture. Thus, some students feel fatigued and easily distracted; others feel heavily scrutinized. The philosopher Evan Selinger (2020) suggests these tendencies are exacerbated by our awareness that they come as the world has been 'shattered and can't be revived'. We are driven, in compensation, to be 'so damned present and empathetic it hurts'.

Besides the difficulties of online education, the history professor Elesha Coffman (2020) claims that the classroom is like live theatre with practical and visible effects. Dreyfus writes that theatre flourishes in a world of film as the direct interaction between performer and audience allows for the active involvement of the spectator, who interactively chooses where to focus. In the theatrical classroom, Coffman writes that students, who see the 'harnesses, wires, pulleys, and pendulums', are drawn into the practice of history and imagine themselves as fellow historians. Videoconferencing, she says, is like CGI, which does not invite participation.

Moltmann and virtual communion

The virtual Eucharist may resemble remote distance education: interpretively difficult, reminiscent of loss, lacking in active participation. This is not necessarily an argument against virtual communion but rather the argument that virtual communion, should it occur, be celebrated in self-conscious awareness of its insufficiency and difficulty. This, however, may be no more than an intensified awareness of absence in 'normal' Eucharists. As Katharine Schmidt (2016) has written, the eucharistic celebration is always suspended between presence and absence as it recalls our distance from God: we intercede for the presence of what cannot be immediate to us.

The 'virtuality' of the virtual Eucharist may intensify three absences that we find described in Moltmann's work. First, the Eucharist is always the celebration of the *entire* church, which can never be physically present. (As Teresa Berger [2018] recounts, Peter Damian allowed even a hermit praying in solitude to use the plural 'us' in the liturgical texts.) At present, our physical celebrations of the Eucharist exclude those who cannot attend, especially those imprisoned. Moltmann (1993a, p. 44) writes that a church that has resigned itself to a 'profane' existing alongside the 'sacred' 'constantly bears with it its own crisis' if it remembers God's identification with the ungodly. In the celebration of a virtual Eucharist, this preexisting 'crisis' becomes hauntingly clear.

Second, the Eucharist is the celebration of the church *in time*. As Moltmann writes, liturgy exists through 'the in-streaming powers of the future power', but with the reminder of the 'qualitative differentiation between past and future' (Moltmann, 2004, pp. 139, 138). We celebrate from a position of incompleteness as we grasp a 'margin' between even our most faithful practice and the coming kingdom (Blevins, 2005), trusting that Christ is present in both the 'form of the crucified Christ' who '"dwells" in this godless world' and 'the form of the Risen Christ' who 'anticipates through the presence of his Spirit' the new creation to come as our world passes away (Moltmann, 2004, p. 267).

A third absence derives from the eternal 'eucharistic sacrifice' within the divine life itself (Moltmann, 1993b). The pandemic reveals a presence-in-absence in congregations and communities, as even in the absence of the Eucharist, the ability to pray through virtually-mediated means allows communities to grow deeper in prayer and connection, while at the same time grieving their physical separation.

Moltmann describes this unity-in-separation as the situation of Jesus on the cross: 'In the cross, Father and Son are most deeply separated in forsakenness and at the same time are most inwardly one in their surrender. What proceeds from this event between Father and Son is the Spirit which justifies the godless, fills the forsaken with love and even brings the dead alive, since even the fact that they are dead cannot exclude them from this event of the cross; the death in God also includes them' (Moltmann, 1993a, p. 244).

The separation in our virtual gatherings points the Church back to the Crucified One. Every Eucharist is a remembering and making present of Christ's sacrifice on the cross; it is Jesus on the cross whose body and blood we share. Thus, the forsaken Christ lends his character of forsakenness to his Eucharistic presence. The element of absence in a virtual Eucharist expresses not only the separation across time and space common to every Eucharist, but also the eschatological reality of the Son's forsakenness which persists eternally—in dialectical tension with the victorious reunion with the Father accomplished through the resurrection—in the divine Trinitarian life. As Moltmann writes, the early twentieth-century Anglican tradition particularly recognized this 'necessity of seeing the eucharistic sacrifice, the cross on Golgotha, and the heart of the triune God together, in a single perspective....The cross on Golgotha has revealed the eternal heart of the Trinity' (Moltmann, 1993b, loc. 552).

Questions

The question for the virtual Eucharist, then, is whether the emphasis on absence still allows for the emergence of what Bishop Doyle describes as 'transcendent reality'. If not, virtual practices may be useful, but as *sacramentals* — similar to interior pilgrimages or devotions before replicas, in which the distinction from the real Jerusalem or the physical grotto at Lourdes is still maintained and significant (Schmidt, 2016). Then, perhaps the distanced bread and wine act only as material signs to aid in making an act of 'spiritual communion' (cf. Anderson, 2020), which proceeds from the realization that the Body of Christ is always in excess of the otherwise inaccessible Eucharistic signs (McGowan, 2020).

However, if the element of absence allows for participation in the 'transcendent reality' of a Trinitarian life characterized by both love and forsakenness, then a virtual Eucharist is the reminder that God is present with us amidst tragedy, existing in tension with the failure of a church perpetually facing the 'crisis' of those excluded and its distance from its eschatological fulfillment. Liturgy, in other words, has always been interpretively difficult, reminiscent of loss, lacking in active participation. The Eucharist, particularly, is itself inherently a making-present of the death of God and the body of Christ who comes to us only in the full scandal of Jesus' abandonment on the cross.

Thus, we suggest that the church's discussion of the virtual Eucharist should not be discernment of the adequacy or normality of virtual life. It is not the search for a Silicon Valley solution. Instead, we should ask whether presence and absence are to be balanced against one another, so that a sufficient level of presence (or acceptable level of absence) is required for the celebration of the Eucharist, or if presence and absence instead exist in a dialectical relationship that reflects an originating dialectic of cross and resurrection in God. The discussion of the virtual Eucharist should take the form of a larger discussion of Moltmann's theology, if in a newly (and urgently) pastoral form.

As we mentioned, we have participated in such a discussion and constructively disagree. Against Moltmann, one can argue that the absence in our time of COVID-19 may be a form of suffering that should lead us to confusion and silence—an acknowledgement of our inarticulacy and what Karen Kilby calls 'something-like-apophasis' (Kilby, 2020, p. 102), our ability to speak only in terms of what cannot be said. Here, our perplexity is dangerously preempted by automatically seeing God in its midst and imagining that our liturgical actions are always on the side of (unseen and likely abstract) victims (Kilby, 2003). For this view, which itself can problematically veer towards a fascination with God's incomprehensibility (Kilby, 2020), this is not a time for a virtual Eucharist amidst physical absence or even a voluntarily accepted spiritual discipline, such as a 'Eucharistic fast', but what Ephraim Radner (2020) has called the acknowledgement of 'famine' and a hope for unforeseeable growth from unimaginable loss.

Conclusion

The question becomes whether a virtual Eucharist is a preemption of the reality of loss, as Dhingra imagines, or if—following Moltmann's theology of the cross—it is the acknowledgement that God's presence only occurs amidst the loss that is always there, as Bowman holds. Did Moltmann's experience of the presence of Jesus in the pre-protest

Virtual Communion, COVID-19, and the Nature of the Body of Christ

Eucharist on the floor of a publisher's office derive from the physical gathering or from the reality of the upcoming practice of solidarity with victims of war—a practice that leaves them no longer simply unseen and abstract? Whatever answer, the question of a virtual Eucharist should point the church's Eucharistic theology, even in 'normal' times, to deeper engagement with the relationship between suffering and sacrament and the reality of God's presence and absence in both.

Hannah Bowman is an M.A. student at Mount St. Mary's University, Los Angeles, California.

Neil Dhingra is a doctoral student at the College of Education, University of Maryland, College Park.

Questions for Discussion

1. What is the theological significance of a sense of absence in our Eucharistic celebrations?

2. Does that absence echo Jesus' forsakenness on the Cross?

3. Would a virtual Eucharist manifest God's presence-in-absence in ways previously unrecognized by us?

References

Anderson, E. (2020). 'Wash your own feet': on singleness and the domestic church [Online]. Available at: https://earthandaltarmag.com/posts/wash-your-own-feet-on-singleness-and-the-domestic-church (Accessed: 28 May 2020).

Berger, T. (2018). *@Worship: Liturgical practices in digital worlds*. New York: Routledge.

Blevins, D. (2005) '"On earth as (if) it is in heaven": Practicing a liturgical eschatology,' *Wesleyan Theological Journal*, 40(1), pp. 69–92.

Bowman, H. (2020). Virtual communion and the call to discern the body [Online]. Available at: https://livingchurch.org/covenant/2020/04/03/virtual-communion-and-the-call-to-discern-the-body/ (Accessed: 23 June 2020).

Coffman, E. (2020). 'Flying by foy in the classroom' [online]. Available at: https://www.patheos.com/blogs/anxiousbench/2020/04/flying-by-foy-in-the-classroom/ (Accessed: 26 May 2020).

Doyle, C. A. (2020). A reflection on the Eucharist during the time of COVID-19: A pastoral letter [online]. Available at: https://28f7fb3fa1a43717a53b-cb342165bfeaa4f2927aec8e5d7de41f.ssl.cf2.rackcdn.com/uploaded/o/0e10076272_1585949934_on-the-eucharist.pdf (Accessed: 26 May 2020).

Dreyfus, H. (2009 [2001]). *On the Internet*. 2nd ed. New York: Routledge.

Kilby, K. (2003). 'Evil and the limits of theology,' *New Blackfriars* 84(983), pp. 13-29.

Kilby, K. (2020). 'Negative theology and meaningless suffering,' *Modern Theology* 36(1), p92-104.

McGowan, A. (2020). Liturgy in a time of plague [online]. Available at: http://abmcg.blogspot.com/2020/03/liturgy-in-time-of-plague.html (Accessed: 26 May 2020).

Moltmann, J. (1993a [1974]) *The Crucified God*. Minneapolis, MN: Fortress.

Moltmann, J. (1993b [1981]) *The Trinity and the Kingdom*. Minneapolis, MN: Fortress. Kindle e-book. (Accessed: 28 May 2020).

Moltmann, J. (2004 [1996]). *The Coming of God*. Minneapolis, MN: Fortress.

Moltmann, J. (2009). *A broad place: An autobiography*. Minneapolis, MN: Fortress.

Radner, E., Martins, D., Dhingra, N. and Hansen, J. (2020). *The Living Church Podcast* [Podcast]. 2 April.

Available at https://anchor.fm/living-church/episodes/In-Retrospect--Will-We-Have-Been-Wise-ec8q9s (Accessed: 1 June 2020).

Reklis, K. (2012). X-Reality and the Incarnation [online]. Available at: http://www.cpx.cts.edu/newmedia/findings/essays/x-reality-and-the-incarnation (Accessed: 26 May 2020).

Rundell, S. (2019). 'Sacraments in digital space—a theological reflection of three churches' position statements,' MA dissertation, Cranmer Hall, St John's College, Durham, UK.

Schmidt, K. (2016). 'Virtual communion: Theology of the internet and the Catholic imagination,' PhD thesis, University of Dayton, Dayton, OH.

Selinger, E. (2020). 'The problem isn't Zoom fatigue' [online]. Available at: https://onezero.medium.com/the-problem-isnt-zoom-fatigue-it-s-mourning-life-as-we-knew-it-5651bf9053a6 (Accessed: 26 May 2020).

Stoddard, A. L. (2020). 'A Eucharistic proposal for a time of pandemic' [online]. Available at: https://www.harvardepiscopalians.org/a-eucharistic-proposal (Accessed: 26 May 2020).

Vernon, M. (2020). 'Zoom fear and Skype fatigue' [online]. Available at: https://www.markvernon.com/zoom-fear-and-skype-fatigue (Accessed: 26 May 2020).

Ward, G. (2020). *Cities of God*. New York: Routledge.

— Pre-Pandemic Ethics —
Triage and Discrimination

Margaret B. Adam and David L. Clough

At the time of writing, parts of the United States are exploding with protests against yet another police killing of a Black man and against the 400 years of systemic oppression, abuse, deprivation, and murder of Black people in a country built on slavery. In response, some British people are calling attention to the United Kingdom's participation in the slave trade and the racial and ethnic discrimination that continues today. Concurrently, the UK COVID-19 death rates are disproportionately high among Black African, Black Caribbean, Bangladeshi, Pakistani, and Indian people in the UK (OFN, 2020; Platt and Warwick, 2020), as well as among care home residents, carers, essential workers, and people living with disabilities and pre-existing conditions. The effects of the pandemic demonstrate the systemic social disparities of life and death in the UK. This is the context in which the authors consider Christian pandemic ethics, and this calls for a shift of focus away from pandemic ethics to what we are calling 'pre-pandemic ethics'.

Earlier in 2020, the authors argued that medical triage in pandemic crisis should aim to save as many lives as possible (Adam and Clough, 2020). When the need for ICU beds and specialised treatments overwhelms the available resources, triage should prioritize the patients most likely to survive and recover with short-term care, while offering palliative care for those who are less likely to survive, or to recover without long-term care. This practice is neither desirable nor supportable except as an emergency measure. Pandemic triage designed to save the most lives accentuates already-prevalent discrimination against those who have the least protection from COVID-19. It perpetuates the privileges of white, wealthy, and healthy people, and increases the vulnerability those in greatest need, thereby reversing the goals of Christian discipleship. 'Christians should be very uncomfortable with any shift from ordinary time ethics to extraordinary time ethics, when that change diminishes the importance of claims previously determined to be essential' (Adam and Clough, 2020). To minimise malign effects, triage should not extend past the pandemic crisis, so that all patients in need can receive live-saving treatment as soon as possible, including those with less promising prognoses. In the present paper, the authors shift their focus from pandemic triage ethics to pre-pandemic ethics: ethics before this pandemic and before the next pandemic. Triage to save the most lives may always be necessary in extreme crises, but pre-pandemic ethics can diminish both the need for triage and the effects of its injustice.

The COVID-19 pandemic is apocalyptic in the popular sense of an unprecedented (in recent history) threat to ordinary life, as in fictional accounts of murderous zombies, alien invasions, and global population decimation. This pandemic is also apocalyptic in the theological sense: it reveals what is ordinarily ignored or unseen. It unveils 'pre-existing systemic human injustices that demand our urgent attention in order to avoid returning to our pre-pandemic complacent acceptance of them' (Clough, 2020). The theological apocalypse of COVID-19 reveals the broken social structures that cause more suffering and death to those already suffering the greatest, and it exposes the agents of that brokenness. Christians who are committed to discipleship must respond to pandemic apocalypse by seeing the brokenness that has been unveiled, and by reversing the hierarchies of privilege.

The COVID-19 pandemic reveals the widespread, pre-existing, preferential treatment of the *least* vulnerable people. Today's challenging dilemmas about who should receive what treatment, protection, and support are the direct result of decisions made long before this pandemic — decisions about which people deserve the most attention, which lives are worth the most, which bodies and capacities are most desirable. Christians have all participated in pre-pandemic ethics: as beneficiaries or victims of discrimination and as stakeholders in and casualties of the ideological distribution of resources. Christians should be gathering together as the Body of Christ to discern responses to the pandemic, with accountability for the past and a focus on changes for the future. Christians should respond to this pandemic and prepare for future crises by prioritising — now — those who are *most* vulnerable. This prioritising requires Christians to recognise that the local and universal manifestations of Christ's body contain within them members who experience more and less advantage, suffer more and less discrimination, and live in more and less precarious conditions. Christians should respond to the COVID-19 apocalypse, as Christians, by recognizing that not all Christians share the same positions of power, agency, and socio-economic security. Those Christians who understand themselves to be representative Christians should be learning from others, in this apocalypse, about the disparity of advantages they have not yet seen. Church communities who follow Jesus Christ's preferential care for those in the greatest need will address the health disparities amongst themselves and beyond, by addressing the social factors that contribute to higher rates of COVID-19 suffering and death among minority populations of the UK. SARS-CoV-2 is a new virus; COVID-19 research has only just begun. But it is already clear that the risk of death is greater for people who are older or live in care homes, who live with disabilities and pre-existing conditions, who are carers, nurses and doctors, who live in poverty, who work in a particular set of occupations, and who are Black, Asian, and minority ethnic (BAME).

> [I]n reality, an ethical approach aimed at maximizing lives saved results in prioritizing certain social groups. The easy lives to save will be those of people who already enjoy social privilege. As a population, younger, white, wealthy people will be more likely to derive benefit from the ICU resources and survive because they enjoy, on average, higher baseline health status.
> (Martín, 2020; see also Ballantyne, 2020)

The SARS-CoV-2 virus has arrived in the midst of a society already formed by the expectation that certain people are more worthy of attention and protection than others. It has become clear that living circumstances before COVID-19 infection strongly influence a patient's likelihood of surviving ICU treatment (ONS, 2020). The people who face the greatest risk of death from the virus are the people most disadvantaged by pre-pandemic decisions and policies. Triage reflects and perpetuates racism, ableism, ageism, and classism (Mastroiani, 2020; Voluntary Health Scotland, 2020). Doctors cannot change the pre-COVID-19 lives of the people who arrive at hospital in need of treatment, but Christians can hold each other accountable for addressing the societal brokenness revealed by the pandemic. Tackling systemic discrimination *before* a pandemic, through community formation, planning, and attention to vulnerabilities, may reduce some of the triage pressure and may render death rates more proportionate across demographics.

It is possible that research will pinpoint genetic differences that contribute to the severity of COVID-19, but there is no non-white race gene to blame; there is no biological common denominator that applies across BAME populations (Morgan, 2020). Instead, BAME people are less likely to be able to work at home, more likely to need public transportation to commute to work, to work in high-contagion conditions, to live in densely populated areas, to experience deprivation and poverty, and less likely to be able to self-isolate. BAME people who disproportionately experience these disadvantages are also less respected at work and in public spheres and less financially stable. They are less likely to be represented in pre-pandemic planning and less likely to be heard when asking for PPE or safer working conditions (Khunti et al., 2020). It was and is no secret that hospitals employ disproportionately large numbers of BAME doctors and nurses, and that doctors and nurses face increased risk of exposure to contagions. These are facts that should warrant extra supplies for protection. And yet, PPE was not readily available when and where needed. 'The first 11 doctors who sadly lost their lives to COVID-19 were all from BAME communities ... ethnic minorities continue to be at the sharp end of the virus and its casualties' (Ali, 2020). Pre-existing discrimination causes increased suffering and death in populations that the dominant ideology cares less about. Christians who hope to see as Christ sees should attend to the breadth of factors that lead to disproportionate COVID-19 deaths in some populations and recognise the radically different contexts in which people experience the pandemic. White congregations should reach out to BAME congregations in humility, to ask if they can listen and learn. BAME congregations should not feel constrained to tell or show white congregations just how damaging their inattentiveness and presumption is.

White Christians have not spent their entire lives coping with the particular social and physical disadvantages experienced daily by BAME people. This lack of experience helps to support white people's belief that COVID-19 is a problem to beat, battle, defeat, or conquer (Reddie, 2020). The fact that COVID-19 may not be conquerable seems difficult to accept for white people with less exposure to persistent, inescapable oppression: '[d]iscrimination and inequalities, whether that's through overcrowded housing, greater risk of health vulnerabilities or economic disadvantage, are a fact of life for Black, Asian, and minority ethnic

(BAME) people in modern Britain' (Unite, 2020). White people who do not appreciate these social realities are tempted to ignore both those at greater risk of death in BAME communities and their wisdom about the systemic causes and effects of health vulnerabilities. Christians should be working together to recognise and serve those in greatest need, and to diminish the causes and effects of disadvantage and increased vulnerability, at both local and policy levels.

Older people are also at increased risk of death from COVID-19: 'over-65s are 34 times more likely to die of coronavirus than working-age Britons' (McIntyre, 2020). Yet, COVID-19 government leaders paid insufficient attention to the pre-pandemic studies calling for the prioritisation of care home residents and care workers. The recommended protective measures did not take place, illustrating

> the widespread social presumption that the lives of elderly people are not as valuable as others... elders in care and their carers currently represent the highest death rates of COVID-19 in the UK; the people who needed the most protection received the least (Lynch and Allamby, 2020; see also Coker, 2020).

The pandemic and the subsequent lockdown have also multiplied the disadvantages and invisibility of those people with disabilities who are already struggling with daily life challenges. '"Underlying health conditions" increasingly feels like a euphemism for those society has quietly given up on' (Ryan, 2020). Christians have a call to meet Jesus in the eyes of their neighbours in need, at each stage of living and dying and in every state of health and dis/ability. Christian communities who spend time and energy building supportive relationships with carers and visiting with those receiving care, know well that older people and people living with disabilities are not expendable. Pre-pandemic research highlighted the heightened dangers for them and their carers; the COVID-19 pandemic confirms those dangers and the malign effects of not preparing for them. Christians should ensure that care home residents, their carers, their families and their church supporters have a place on crisis planning committees, to share their wisdom, and to make it more difficult for the general public to ignore and neglect them in plans for future crises.

Christians should be dismantling unjust social structures now—within this pandemic and before the next—to illustrate the hope of Christ: that the reconciliation of creation renders oppression neither necessary nor justifiable. In this life, there may always be a scarcity of supplies in unprecedented crises, but churches should be planning now for the protection and nurturing of vulnerable people. And Christians should now be redistributing the resources of healthy, wealthy, and white Christians, so that no one will face the next pandemic without social protection and security. There is no clearer proclamation of the work of Christ in the world than prioritising those with the fewest advantages. This is what Christians need to be doing now.

Margaret B. Adam is Postdoctoral Researcher for the three-year, AHRC-funded project: Christian Ethics of Farmed Animal Welfare, and Visiting Tutor in Ethics at St Stephen's House, Oxford.

David L. Clough is Professor of Theological Ethics at University of Chester and the Principal Investigator of the Christian Ethics of Farmed Animal Welfare project. He is also Visiting Professor at the Centre for Animal Welfare, University of Winchester.

Questions for Discussion

1. In what ways is your church community responsible for the disproportionately damaging effects of COVID-19 on those people who are already disadvantaged? In what ways does the responsibility lie elsewhere?

2. What might you and your community do now to prepare for the discriminatory effects of ongoing and future pandemics?

References

Adam, M. and Clough, D. (2020). 'Christian ethics and the dilemma of triage during a pandemic', *ABC Religion and Ethics*, 16 April [online]. Available at: https://www.abc.net.au/religion/christian-ethics-and-the-dilemma-of-triage-during-a-pandemic/12146944 (Accessed: 2 June 2020).

Aldridge, R. W. et al. (2020). 'Black, Asian and Minority Ethnic groups in England are at increased risk of death from COVID-19: indirect standardisation of NHS mortality data', *Wellcome Open Research*, 6 May [online]. Available at: https://wellcomeopenresearch.org/articles/5-88 (Accessed: 2 June 2020).

Ali, S. (2020). 'BAME life chances, Covid inequality and death', *Green World*, 6 May [online]. Available at: https://greenworld.org.uk/

article/bame-life-chances-covid-inequality-and-death (Accessed 2 June 2020).

Ballantyne, A. (2020). 'ICU triage: How many lives or whose lives?' *Journal of Medical Ethics Blog*, 7 April [online]. Available at: https://blogs.bmj.com/medical-ethics/2020/04/07/icu-triage-how-many-lives-or-whose-lives/ (Accessed 2 June 2020).

Brown, R. et al. (2020). 'Is ethnicity linked to incidence or outcomes of covid-19?', *British Medical Journal*, 369, m1548 [online]. Available at: https://www.bmj.com/content/369/bmj.m1548/rr-6?fbclid=IwAR0LinVPCr20eEaz7bHh3h4LsaSM-uOC6Cr5SC-zVJkTZKIwdCSaXR1zqgI (Accessed 2 June 2020)

Clough, D. (2020). 'Pandemic as Animal Apocalypse', paper for the Cambridge Senior Seminar in Christian Theology, May.

Coker, R. (2020). 'Harvesting' is a terrible word – but it's what has happened in Britain's care homes', *The Guardian*, 8 May [online]. Available at: https://www.theguardian.com/commentisfree/2020/may/08/care-home-residents-harvested-left-to-die-uk-government-herd-immunity (Accessed 2 June 2020).

Khunti, K. et al., (2020). 'Preliminary signals must be explored urgently', *British Medical Journal*, 369, m1548 [online]. Available at https://www.bmj.com/content/369/bmj.m1548 (Accessed: 2 June 2020).

Lynch, E., Allamby, L., (2020), *Commissioner for Older People for Northern Ireland News*, 7 May [online]. Available at: https://www.copni.org/news/2020/may/article-by-eddie-lynch-commissioner-for-older-people-for-northern-ireland-and-les-allamby-chief-commissioner-northern-ireland-human-rights-commission (Accessed: 2 June 2020).

Martín, I. (2020). '"Slum bishop" of Buenos Aires says pandemic exposes pre-existing injustice', *Crux*, 21 May [online]. Available at: https://cruxnow.com/covid-19/2020/05/slum-bishop-of-buenos-aires-says-pandemic-exposes-pre-existing-injustice/ (Accessed: 2 June 2020).

Mastroiani, J. (2020). '"Real People Won't Die": Rhetoric around who is at risk of coronavirus infection sparks debate over ageism, ableism', *National Post*, 3 March [online]. Available at: https://nationalpost.com/news/world/real-people-wont-die-why-the-rhetoric-around-who-is-at-risk-for-coronavirus-is-so-harmful (Accessed: 2 June 2020).

McIntyre, N. (2020). 'Pensioners 34 times more likely to die of Covid-19 than working age Brits, data shows', *The Guardian*, 13 May [online]. Available at: https://www.theguardian.com/uk-news/2020/may/13/pensioners-34-times-more-likely-to-die-of-covid-19-than-working-age-brits-data-shows (Accessed: 2 June 2020).

Morgan, W. (2020). 'Coronavirus: Its impact cannot be explained away through the prism of race', *The Conversation*, 28 May [online]. Available at: https://theconversation.com/coronavirus-its-impact-cannot-be-explained-away-through-the-prism-of-race-138046 (Accessed: 2 June 2020).

Office for National Statistics (2020). 'Coronavirus (COVID-19) related deaths by ethnic group, England and Wales: 2 March 2020 to 15 May 2020', 19 June [online]. Available at: https://www.ons.gov.uk/peoplepopulationandcommunity/birthsdeathsandmarriages/deaths/articles/relateddeathsbyethnicgroupenglandandwales/2march-2020to10april2020 (Accessed: 30 June 2020).

Patel, H. (2020). '"Reckoning" needed on disproportionate Covid-19 deaths amongst black and Pakistani and Bangladeshi heritage people', Unite, 7 May [online]. Available at: https://unitetheunion.org/news-events/news/2020/may/reckoning-needed-on-disproportionate-covid-19-deaths-amongst-black-and-pakistani-and-bangladeshi-heritage-people (Accessed: 2 June 2020).

Platt, L. and Warwick, R. (2020). 'Are Some Ethnic Groups More Vulnerable to COVID-19 than Others?' Institute of Fiscal Studies, 1 May [online]. Available at: https://www.ifs.org.uk/publications/14827 (Accessed: 2 June 2020).

Reddie, A. G. (2020). In discussion during 'The Ethical Challenges of Covid-19' a webinar sponsored by The Centre for Baptist Studies, Regent's Park College, Oxford University, 18 May.

Royal College of Psychiatrists (2020). 'Impact of COVID-19 on Black, Asian and Minority Ethnic (BAME) staff in mental healthcare settings | assessment and management of risk', 13 May [online]. Available at: https://www.rcpsych.ac.uk/docs/default-source/about-us/covid-19/impact-of-covid19-on-bame-staff-in-mental-healthcare-settings_assessment-and-management-of-risk_13052020v2.pdf?sfvrsn=1068965_2 (Accessed 2 June 2020).

Ryan, F. (2020). 'Coronavirus has made it even easier to forget about disabled people', Guardian, 29 April [online]. Available at: https://www.theguardian.com/commentisfree/2020/apr/29/coronavirus-disabled-people-inequality-pandemic (Accessed: 2 June 2020).

Voluntary Health Scotland (2020). 'COVID-19: A pandemic in the age of inequality', 7 May [online]. Available at: https://vhscotland.org.uk/covid-19-a-pandemic-in-the-age-of-inequality/ (Accessed: 2 June 2020).

Book Reviews

Theological Reflection: Methods
Elaine Graham, Heather Walton and Frances Ward,
SCM, 2019, iv + 300 pp., pbk, £25.99

The production of a second edition of *Theological Reflection: Methods* raises the question of how far the teaching and practice of theological reflection has developed, or not, in the past fourteen years. The revised Introduction to this work suggests that despite the proliferation of theory on the subject and its being increasingly embedded in theological education, the danger of shallow and ill-informed practice remains a persistent issue. (1-2) The main purpose of this second edition and its most salutary aspect is not, however, to labour this point, but rather to bring its material up to date with recent developments in theology, society and culture, so that it remains a practical and relevant resource for students, teachers and practitioners in theology, ministry and mission.

Adopting the scheme of 'methods' rather than 'models', Graham, Walton and Ward address theological reflection in a manner that requires critical and imaginative engagement on the part of the reader. As such it works best as a teaching resource or as a higher-level introduction, rather than as a step by step 'how to' of theological reflection. Broadly speaking, it introduces theology-as-process through the lens of practical theology, by asking the important question: 'What if all theology were approached as if it were practical theology?' (9) This approach makes the book particularly attractive for those concerned with practical ministry and mission as it illustrates how theologians throughout history, from St Paul to Margery Kempe to Karl Barth to Rebecca Chopp, construct theology in and for a particular context, and for the threefold purpose of Christian formation, edifying the church and communicating with the world.

The specific contribution of these three scholars to the field of practical theology in the last decade has been substantial, and

Book Reviews

is brought to bear on this work. Chapter 1, 'Theology by Heart' discusses the work of Ward on lifelong learning (37-41) and Walton on spiritual life writing (44-47), while chapter five, 'Speaking of God in Public' includes a section on Graham's work on apologetics (177-180). The updated material is at points tilted towards their particular methodological interests, such as chapter 1, which covers Walton's concern with theopoetics and trauma theology through the work of Shelly Rambo. (79-83) However the approach overall ensures that a diversity of perspectives are covered.

Each chapter is laid out in a common structure, and while the earlier sections, covering scriptural and historical foundations, remain substantially the same, there have been significant revisions to the latter section which covers the contemporary application of each method. Chapter 1, for example, takes account of how technological change affects the practice of journaling, through the 'spiritual blogging' of Nadia Bolz-Weber. (47-50) Chapter 3, 'Telling God's Story', covers John Swinton's work on disability and hospitality. (111-114) Chapter 4, 'Writing the Body of Christ', engages with mission-shaped church and the fresh expressions initiative in the Church of England as well as the development of new monasticism. (144-7) Chapter 6, 'Theology-In-Action', goes beyond liberation theology to explore Ray Gaston's work on interfaith relations. (208-212) Chapter 7, 'Theology in the Vernacular', replaces Robert Beckford with James H. Cone as a representative of black theology, and includes Marcella Althaus-Reid's work on queering theology. (236-243) These are by and large are well chosen additions that help the reader to engage with issues of contemporary concern for church and society.

The 'Evaluation' section to each chapter has in many cases been sharpened to consider more incisively the benefits and pitfalls of each method in contemporary contexts and iterations. The final 'Questions' section has been replaced by a critical bibliography of 'Further Reading', which encourages a broader and deeper range of further engagement than previously. Each bibliography offers enticing critical introductions to a range of classic and contemporary works. The former, such as Bonhoeffer's *Letters and Papers*, may be of particular interest to students, the latter, such as the work of Courtney T. Goto and Zoë Bennett, of more interest to theological educators. While the final chapter is devoted to 'contextual' theologies, there is reference to texts and theologians from a range of cultures and contexts throughout the book, as well as close attention paid to gender balance and inclusivity throughout.

For those who found the first edition a useful resource, this second edition is a worthwhile update. It will ensure that this continues to be a key text for those in ministry, mission and theological education for years to come.

Beth Dod, Sarum College

Christian hospitality and Muslim Immigration in an Age of Fear

Matthew Kaemingk,
Eerdamans, 2018, viii + 338 pp., pbk, £14.89

Matthew Kaemingk teaches at Fuller Theological Seminary, and writes out of a background of Dutch Calvinism but with broad sympathies and a subtle ear for contemporary discourses concerning how western societies can stay recognisably democratic as the present century grows weirder. Having spent time researching in the Netherlands for this project, the book speaks more clearly to the European reader than some ethical expositions from the heartlands of enlightened American evangelicalism. This Dutch experience, as the grip of a liberal modernism has given way to confusion and to openings for the far right, in the face of social changes for whose complexity the number of Muslim immigrants stands proxy, is really quite helpful as a benchmark against which to assess the currents of thought and political choosing in Britain.

The book's title gives a clue as to its beginning and ending but not so much the 200 pages which are the meat of it: they hold a careful exposition of a Christian position on pluralism. This is very useful, because while everyone agrees that multiculturalism is old hat no one is quite sure what should be taking its place. The author describes how in the Netherlands in the 1960s and thereafter the language of extreme tolerance disguised an actual hegemony of secular liberalism, abetted by a willingness of the Protestant academy to secularise its theology and ethics in large measure. He then reaches back towards the towering figure of Abraham Kuyper (1827-1920), the Calvinist Christian leader who eventually became Prime Minister of the Netherlands. Some readers will flinch at this name. Does not Kuyper represent a hegemonic Calvinism, an assertion of the sovereignty of Christ over absolutely every sphere of life? Are we being dragged back to sixteenth century Geneva? No. Carefully and quite elegantly, Kaemingk sets out a case for 'Christian pluralism' on the basis of exploration of Kuyper's scattered writings: a useful service, since Kuyper did not produce a single exposition of his public theology. Although it becomes almost homiletic at times, the strongest part of the book is the setting out of a positive understanding of social plurality as a good, setting it in contrast to various forms of tyranny of the majority or of an elite. Christology, the 'hospitality of the Cross', eschatology and many other core theological themes support the argument in quite a powerful way. The perspective is definitely ecclesial, and includes a strong if not startlingly original chapter on 'pluralism and worship'. One of its attractive features is that he forswears any attempt to set out a systematic vision of what a plural society should look like: in the sharing of 'common grace, a common humanity, and a common creation ... a real hope that moments of moral consensus and cooperation can be found' (155): in an eschatological context, such milestones are sufficient.

A reader who borrowed this book and did not have leisure to come to grips with its theological ethics could nevertheless gain much from its first part, a case study of the Netherlands in recent history and today, and the final 75 pages which focus on the scope for Christian action. While the author does not quite have the authenticity of someone who has lived the reality of urban areas with high ethnic minority and immigrant populations, he has talked at length to many who do so live, and their testimony of incarnational service, witness and growth in humility comes through strongly. One of the best potential uses of this book is in subverting baldly conversionist, stereotyping and demonising attitudes toward Muslims; the history of this in white evangelical America since 1990 (Muslims gradually replacing Russia as the foe to unite against) is well and in no way shrilly set out. The book concludes, in fact, with ten specific pointers for Christian responses to Islam in America.

As an evangelical the author is of course not against Christian witness to Muslims, and is writes well on how converts from Islam are a blessing to the church in changing it; but he is also free with examples of how those of different faiths living alongside one another especially in the context of hospitality, are a present blessing to each other and to their communities. In the end his practical prescription centres round a simple vision of faith communities developing trust and ease with one another through sewing, eating, sharing everyday life together. These stories are encouraging, and are more fully told in other places than this book; Kaemingk's contribution is to do justice to the Spirit's work in neighbourliness, while setting it without tweeness or artificiality in a robust framework of Protestant theological ethics.

Martin Kettle, associate inspector HM Inspectorate of Prisons

The Dangers of Christian Practice

Lauren Winner
Yale University Press, 2018, 230pp., hbk, £18.00

This is a captivating read: Lauren Winner draws on a wealth of insight, and a variety of historical and liturgical exemplars, to illustrate her central thesis about Christian practices. That is, that they are themselves often deformed and impaired, just as much as any other human customs and symbolic traditioned actions, such that their effect can be lessened. However, Winner goes even further, to describe what she calls "characteristic damage": that which is intrinsic to a thing, proper to it, and not merely incidental. As she puts it: 'What I am after in this book are the damages done to, via, and by the agents of Christian practice, that are about the practices…It is the aim of this book to suggest that deformations of Christian practices are part of the practices themselves…' (16)

She proceeds, after a thoughtful, careful and illuminating opening chapter, to make her case by use of three illustrative examples. Chapter two focuses on the Eucharist, and in particular on the ways in which anti-Jewish feeling and violence have historically found their origins and expression because of it. This is because, she claims, the Eucharistic mystery is at its heart the reception of the Jewish flesh and blood of Christ by Gentile believers. The dissonance this fosters provokes, in part, a reactionary consequence. The following chapter looks at prayer, and focuses on the particular prayers of Keziah Goodwin Hopkins Brevard, as recorded in her 1860 diary. Brevard was an American slave owner, and the force of her intercessions to God is to wish for the improvement of the poor behaviour of her slaves without reference to the sinfulness, evident to us if not to her, of her owning them in the first place, or opening herself to what God's will might be in her situation. Winner proceeds to offer other illustrations of the same principle, and to contrast this with the kinds of prayers

Book Reviews

which are thought eligible to appear in anthologies and collections. It's clear that something is amiss in the ways in which prayer is often understood, utilised and embraced by 'ordinary' Christians: and Winner is astute enough to ponder what similar 'deformations' might occur in contemporary prayer practices.

A third chapter takes baptism as its theme, examining the practice of private baptism, in family homes and without attendant congregations. Here is another piece of damage: a rite intended to signify entry into the life of Christian discipleship and the fellowship of the Church diminished so as merely to effect a welcome to one family for one isolated child. Here in particular, many clergy will find echoes of their own experience, and the frequent dilemmas of how to maintain baptismal authenticity and integrity in the face of families, both churched and unchurched, for whom it represents something rather more domesticated. The requests for effectively 'private' baptisms are a common experience: how then to resist the 'deformation' and renew the practice?

The book is well-written, engaging, lively and thoughtful, and Winner writes with the clear commitment of one for whom the practices she describes matter greatly in the inculcation of faith and the cultivation of devotion. She also, in the final section, offers characteristically hopeful and positive assessments of the ways in which such 'damaged' practices can both still be effective and be 'repristinated'. She does so without ever refusing to deal with the realities she describes and the import of what she relates. It's possible, for all that, that the book is less successful in two key areas. Firstly, it's not always clear, especially after the chapter on the Eucharist, that Winner quite makes the case for the "characteristic damage" she claims in each case, beyond the general (but not unimportant!) claim that all things are affected by human sinfulness. Secondly, her focus is sometimes too narrow. This is naturally unavoidable in a thesis with a scope and implications as wide as this, but it does tend at times to a rather reductionist proposition. For instance, much more needs to be said about the ways in which the Eucharist is and has been 'damaged' than simply to examine medieval anti-Jewishness, and its effect on future generations. And much more also needs to be said about the sin of anti-Jewishness itself, besides the ways in which it has sometimes been manifest in Eucharistic thought and practice. Likewise, the ways in which prayer is deformed and damaged by sin are manifold and severe, and the brief chapter here can only scratch the surface.

For all that, this is a compelling and engrossing read, which raises vital questions and stimulates urgent enquiry and reflection about the relationship between practice and faith, liturgy and belief, piety and discipleship. It represents an important call for critical awareness and spiritual re-formation in much of our Christian devotional life.

Jonathan Dean, Methodist Church House

Food and Faith, A Theology of Eating

Norman Wirzba,
CUP, 2019, xx + 319, pbk, £18.59

This book actually changed my life; a dramatic statement but it has moved me from being a somewhat stealthy flexitarian to an outright vegetarian. So I am offering you a trigger warning, it may do the same for you. Stanley Hauerwas had a similar reaction in his Foreword to this book which he found "somewhat painful" to read. (ix) He also 'did not want to know much of what [he] learned by reading this book.' I agree; but I cannot now un-know it. As Gilbert T. Rowe Distinguished Professor of Theology at Duke Divinity School and Director of a major research project entitled 'Facing the Anthropocene', Wirzba is well placed to write on food, faith and how we eat. The fact that this book is in its second edition testifies to its importance as a book for our time.

Wirzba explains in the Preface that the book develops a theological exploration of eating. He explains that what food is and why eating matters is best framed in terms of the 'Trinitarian life of gift and sacrifice, hospitality and communion, care and celebration.' (xi) What we eat, where we eat, how we eat and with whom we eat all matters. A meal is not a random assortment of ingredients nor fuel to keep us going. No, food is a basic expression of God's provision and care and Wirzba claims that when we are mindful of God in our eating, then we are in collaboration with God in God's own original sharing of life.

The book is theological in scope with respect to food and eating. Wirzba deals with themes such as garden, sin, sacrifice, Eucharist, hospitality (a personal favourite), reconciliation and communion. All these are dealt with accessibly and he offers some lovely practical outworkings. He declares that in a world driven and upheld by market forces where those of us in urban centres are becoming increasingly removed from the growth and production of food, we need to reclaim the sacramental sense of life and to receive food as a precious gift. He reminds us that we Christians have much to learn from other religions and indigenous peoples, especially with respect to their relationship with the land.

The book covers much from our identity born in a garden, why eating is a moral and theological issue and some of its malfunctions, the costly nature of creaturely life, the role and purpose of Eucharistic eating, the importance of hospitality, gratitude and celebration and whether there will be eating in heaven. There is a fascinating Epilogue which addresses the question of faithful eating. There is so much gold in here, I can only offer you a few nuggets.

Wirzba's opening gambit reminds us of our interconnectedness with the world. Instead of 'you are what you eat' he reframes this (referring to Michael Pollan) as 'you are what what you eat eats too.' Think about that for a moment. Eating is the constant reminder that we are never alone and that we need to attend to the creatures that nurture us. He claims that with today's food systems we find ourselves in a state of divorce with the world. We are in a relationship of contract, rather than of covenant; a relationship that wants efficiency, convenience and affordability rather than one than honours gift and grace as a way of life. He compares the history of industrial agriculture to industrial architecture using the modernist designs of le Corbusier as an egregious example. This is the heritage that has brought us to this state of divorce, not only metaphorically but also divorced from or oblivious to the contexts in which we live.

Wirzba asserts that eating joins people to one another and 'introduces us to a graced world of hospitality' (41), I love that idea! He explains why bread is so important to us, the comforting smell of a fresh loaf to share together with a companion, *com* (with) *panis* (bread). Friendship is an embodied state of sharing together. He asserts that eating together is a spiritual exercise as we become more attentive to one another and to the world. Gardening is treated in a similar manner and is likened to a spiritual discipline.

He explores the dark side of how our food is produced and how we are now eating in exile because our industrial food culture is one of 'injustice, estrangement and bewilderment.' (113). This is a powerful chapter that considers what it means to live in an exilic eating condition, the most extreme forms of which are manifested in eating disorders. He also acknowledges that God created a world that lives through the eating of its members. This is challenging for the vegetarian as we are slowly learning that plants' lives are more complex than we ever imagined. Or as I like to think of it, 'trees are people too' with the arrogance of a human being! The chapter on Eucharistic eating concludes with an example from the South Side of Chicago where Monica concludes that fresh and healthy food is a civil rights issue and that communion is not a sideshow but the very enactment of life. Wirzba notes how, as a Western culture, we are obsessed with cooking programmes but claim we do not have time to cook. He claims that cooking is one of the fundamental activities that defines us as human beings.

I thoroughly recommend this book. As a New Zealander, I still have a childhood hankering for roast lamb and this has been our Christmas staple since our arrival in the UK 15 years ago, part patriotism, part desire. This last Christmas, to the laughter and astonishment of our carnivorous sons I also made a nut roast! They grudgingly admitted that they liked it. Perhaps change is in the air.

Cathy Ross, CMS, Oxford

Biotechnology, human nature, and Christian ethics

Gerald McKenny,
CUP, 2018, xix + 215 pp., hbk, £75

McKenny's volume arises from the task of Christian ethics to evaluate and respond to an increasing range of new possibilities emerging out of technological progress. The central question he addresses in this context is whether there is a normative human nature which can inform ethical responses to such changes. It is not a question of technology simply enhancing human characteristics but of changing the characteristics themselves.

McKenny's work recognises that contemporary ethical questions in this field are distinctive for their impact rather than their novelty. Human beings have interfered in their nature for a long time; the new challenges come with the scale and accessibility of change.

The book is divided into five chapters, followed by a conclusion. After introducing the key questions under examination, and setting out his view that a normative status for human nature matters to Christian ethics, the following four chapters offer critical evaluations of claims that human nature is normative. This involves grouping various contributions into the categories of human nature as given; as the ground for good and rights; as being open to intervention; and as a nature given in order to relate to God. McKenny concludes with an appendix which explores the intriguing question of what it might mean if change became so radical that we cannot say with confidence that 'someone' is human: that, instead, they are posthuman.

Given the scale and depth of change now possible with biotechnology (or on the horizon) the question of how Christian ethics responds is clearly relevant. The author rightly observes that what may appear to be a technically defined field of study is intimately related to question about society and contemporary politics. This book is a contribution to this task and it does not claim to be exhaustive.

For those unfamiliar, or only slightly acquainted with this topic, it is demanding and rewarding read. It takes us beyond the headline news of a particular development and questions what it may, or may not mean, to hold a belief in a normative human nature. At the end of the book, reflecting on theological considerations, the intriguing question arises about potential posthuman life and Christian faith. If Christ becoming human created the potential for human beings to encounter God in a particular way, would this relationship be available to posthumans?

McKenny is careful not to provide analysis or answers which lack nuance. In this complex territory he is an able guide and assists the reader to understand the issues and questions biotechnology raises. Reading this book led me to reflect on the whole notion of what it means to define normative human nature and how that is determined.

Christopher Swift, Methodist Homes (MHA)

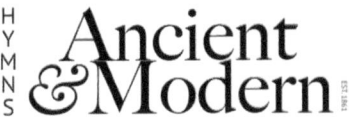

The Canterbury Dictionary of
HYMNOLOGY

The result of over ten years of research by an international team of editors, The Canterbury Dictionary of Hymnology is the major online reference work on hymns, hymn-writers and traditions.

www.hymnology.co.uk

CHURCH TIMES The Church Times, founded in 1863, has become the world's leading Anglican newspaper. It offers professional reporting of UK and international church news, in-depth features on faith, arts and culture, wide-ranging comment and all the latest clergy jobs. Available in print and online.

www.churchtimes.co.uk

Crucible Crucible is the Christian journal of social ethics. It is produced quarterly, pulling together some of the best practitioners, thinkers, and theologians in the field. Each issue reflects theologically on a key theme of political, social, cultural, or environmental significance.

www.cruciblejournal.co.uk

JLS Joint Liturgical Studies offers a valuable contribution to the study of liturgy. Each issue considers a particular aspect of liturgical development, such as the origins of the Roman rite, Anglican Orders, welcoming the Baptised, and Anglican Missals.

www.jointliturgicalstudies.co.uk

magnet Magnet is a resource magazine published three times a year. Packed with ideas for worship, inspiring artwork and stories of faith and justice from around the world.

www.ourmagnet.co.uk

For more information on these publications visit the websites listed above or contact **Hymns Ancient & Modern:**
Tel.: **+44 (0)1603 785 910**
Write to: Subscriptions, Hymns Ancient & Modern,
13a Hellesdon Park Road, Norwich NR6 5DR

CHEQUE OR CREDIT CARD	DIRECT DEBIT
Individual rate UK: ☐ £22	☐ £20
Institutional rate UK: ☐ £30	☐ £28
International rate: ☐ £40	☐ £35
Individual copy ☐ £7	

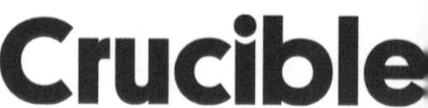

Please complete section 1. Cheque **or** 2. Credit/Debit card **or** 3. Direct debit
(the name and address you give must match the information on your credit/Debit card/bank statement.)

YOUR DETAILS (Please complete)

Title ....Christian name ....Surname ....

Address: ....

....

....

Postcode .... Daytime telephone no ....

Email: ....

- I enclose a cheque for the total amount of £..............
  payable to Hymns Ancient and Modern Ltd.
- To pay by credit/debit card please visit www.crucible.hymnsam.co.uk/subscriptions or contact us on 01603 785911

Ancient & Modern

Instruction to your bank or building society to pay by Direct Debit

DIRECT Debit

Please fill in the whole form using a ball point pen and send to:
Hymns Ancient & Modern Ltd.

Name and full postal address of your bank or building society

To: The Manager Bank/building society

Address

Postcode

Name(s) of account holder(s)

Bank/building society account number

Branch sort code

Service user number

| 2 | 4 | 3 | 2 | 3 | 3 |

Reference

Instruction to your bank or building society
Please pay Hymns Ancient & Modern Ltd Direct Debits from the account detailed in this Instruction subject to the safeguards assured by the Direct Debit Guarantee. I understand that this Instruction may remain with Hymns Ancient & Modern Ltd and, if so, details will be passed electronically to my bank/building society.

Hymns Ancient & Modern Ltd. 13a Hellesdon Park Road, Norwich NR6 5DR

Signature(s)

Banks and building societies may not accept Direct Debit Instructions for some types of account.

This Guarantee should be detached and retained by the payer.

The Direct Debit Guarantee

- This Guarantee is offered by all banks and building societies that accept instructions to pay Direct Debits
- If there are any changes to the amount, date or frequency of your Direct Debit Hymns Ancient & Modern Ltd will notify you 10 working days in advance of your account being debited or as otherwise agreed. If you request Hymns Ancient & Modern Ltd to collect payment, confirmation of the amount and date will be given to you at the time of the request
- If an error is made in the payment of your Direct Debit, by Hymns Ancient & Modern Ltd or your bank or building society, you are entitled to a full and immediate refund of the amount paid from your bank or building society
  - If you receive a refund you are not entitled to, you must pay it back when Hymns Ancient & Modern Ltd asks you to
- You can cancel a Direct Debit at any time by simply contacting your bank or building society. Written confirmation may be required. Please also notify us

www.ingramcontent.com/pod-product-compliance
Ingram Content Group UK Ltd.
Pitfield, Milton Keynes, MK11 3LW, UK
UKHW030902050526
12271UKWH00017B/175